ADDICTION
IS
ADDICTION

Understanding the disease in oneself
and others for a better quality of life

— by —
Raju Hajela
Sue Newton
Paige Abbott

◆ FriesenPress

Suite 300 - 990 Fort St
Victoria, BC, Canada, V8V 3K2
www.friesenpress.com

ISBN
978-1-4602-6644-1 (Hardcover)
978-1-4602-6645-8 (Paperback)
978-1-4602-6646-5 (eBook)

1. Self-Help, Substance Abuse & Addictions

Distributed to the trade by The Ingram Book Company

Table of Contents

Acknowledgements

We are thankful to all the patients and their families who have taught us so much about the disease of Addiction and recovery. It is a privilege to be part of so many people's journeys and witness the transformation of those who embrace recovery.

We appreciate all the contributions of leaders, researchers and clinicians in Addiction Medicine such as Eliot Gardner, Mark Gold, George Koob, Nora Volkow, Ken Blum, Robert Dupont, Abraham Twerski, Stan Gitlow, Stu Gitlow, Mike Miller, Ken Roy, Howard Wetsman, and the many others who have contributed greatly to our growing understanding of various aspects of Addiction. The definition of Addiction that has become the national and international standard was developed through the American Society of Addiction Medicine's Descriptive and Diagnostic Terminology Action Group (DDTAG), which has had numerous contributors under the broad leadership of Mike Miller, Raju Hajela, and Richard Saitz.

We are thankful to Paul Abbott, who was the first to read and edit our book. His feedback and comments were invaluable as he helped us become more deliberate in our messaging.

A special thank you to Dr. Stephen Karpman for granting us permission to use the Karpman Drama Triangle in our text, which we have adapted to explain some important issues related to the dysfunctional traps that can be present in relationships, and develop constructs related to dealing with the dysfunctions.

Introduction

Our goal in writing this book is to increase awareness and understanding of Addiction as a brain disease and quash the notion that it is a moral failing or personal weakness. In time, we hope that there will be more acceptance and compassion for those struggling with active Addiction rather than stigma. We hope people will one day get the necessary treatment and support they need to get into and stay in recovery. This book is written for those who are interested in learning more about Addiction; whether that is for you, a friend, or family member. It is also written for health care providers who want to better understand their patients or clients and who may have been impacted by Addiction in their personal lives.

Addiction is a word that means different things to different people. It is a term most commonly associated with psychoactive or mood altering substances (alcohol and drugs), where a person uses the substance of choice to excess, and it then takes precedence over all other aspects of their lives. Some people use the word in reference to something that a person enjoys doing often and sometimes to excess, generating the comment 'I'm addicted to...' There is an assumption that Addiction is just about problem behaviour and that addictive behaviour is a personal choice. In reality, Addiction is an insidious and powerful disease that takes control over a person's life, creating a significant amount of pain and despair for the person affected, and for those around them.

Many argue that using drugs or alcohol is a choice and a person chooses to become intoxicated episodically or continuously. The negative consequences that may result from intoxication are blamed on making bad choices. While this can be the case with substance abuse, where there may be choice to initiate the use of a substance or engage in addictive behaviour, no one ever chooses to become addicted. We will talk more about substance abuse, which is an old concept that is increasingly being replaced by that of unhealthy substance use that consists of: hazardous use (episodic), harmful use (more continuous) and Addiction, which is characterized by impairment in behavioural control, among other symptoms.

With Addiction, the choice is gone. When the genetic predisposition is strong, even the initiation of substance use is not necessarily done by choice. Losing the ability to make healthy choices in Addiction means that, despite one's best intentions, the problem behaviours persist and aggravate the disease. It becomes important to pay attention to one's behaviours so that changes can be introduced that promote recovery. Focusing on controlling behaviours can serve to aggravate them, whereas attention to building up healthier behaviours reinforces recovery. For example, it can be more beneficial to focus on developing a social network through activities, journaling, meditating, and physical activity than spending energy trying to stop drinking alcohol.

In active Addiction, the pattern that starts to emerge is the need for more, and there is no off switch. Addiction becomes an ever-increasing desire that can never be fulfilled. The chase for more and the preoccupation to fulfill this persistent desire becomes the most important aspect of a person's life. All other responsibilities are neglected and daily life starts to unravel and become increasingly unmanageable. This pattern can occur with any behaviour, including, but not limited to: alcohol, drugs, food, sex, relationships, gambling, video games, shopping, exercise, and work.

One characteristic of the disease of more, or Addiction, is the inability to consistently abstain. An individual may be able to put the compulsive behaviour on hold, but they have difficulty maintaining the abstention and so the behaviour continues over a long period, progressively getting worse. For example, Joan recognizes she has an issue with gambling. Once she starts, she cannot stop until she has lost all her money. One day she decides to stop going to the casino. After a few weeks, she feels irritable and stressed so she goes back to the casino for relief from these feelings. Once she starts gambling again, she again cannot stop and the compulsive behaviour continues.

With Addiction, there can also be impaired control over other behaviours. For example, Joe meets his friends at the bar. The others all have one or two beers and go home, but he drinks to get drunk and consumes nine beers. This occurs fairly regularly, and not only does he have difficulty moderating his intake, others notice that he is unable to follow through on time commitments and responsibilities.

Many people with Addiction have cravings so powerful that they are unable to abstain consistently, despite negative consequences in their life. The desire for more takes priority over everything else in their life, much to the horror and dismay of others.

Typically, those in active Addiction have a diminished recognition of problems in their own behaviour, which is often called denial. They also have problems in relationships. There can be lots of rationalization and minimization of their compulsive behaviours. The person with Addiction may become defensive when challenged by others, or come up with all sorts of excuses and reasons to justify their substance use or behaviours.

Lastly, people with Addiction have a dysfunctional emotional response, meaning that they do not deal with their feelings on a regular basis or in a healthy way. Feelings build up over time until they feel anger or completely shut down. The feelings become too overwhelming and there is an increased desire to numb and escape.

In Chapter 1, we explain what makes Addiction a primary, chronic brain disease. Addiction is influenced by both genetics and environment, similar to other chronic diseases such as diabetes. Simply put, a disease is a malfunction of an organ and is typically manifested by distinguishing symptoms and characteristics. With Addiction, that organ is the brain. All of us are hardwired with reward circuitry in our midbrain that is designed to control our appetites for food and sex. We need food to survive and sex to procreate, and the human brain is designed to make these pleasurable. Anytime something feels good, there is a release of the neurotransmitter dopamine, among others, which makes it more likely we will engage in that behaviour again. Each of us is vulnerable to Addiction because of genetics, brain function, environment, and exposure to substances and unhealthy behaviours.

In Chapter 2, we discuss the historical and current perspectives of Addiction and the birth of its definition (found in Appendix A). There continues to be many viewpoints and inconsistencies in treating Addiction, and historically the focus has been on behaviours and substances. In 2012, the American Society of Addiction Medicine (ASAM) approved a definition of Addiction based on extensive review of current scientific work, lessons learned by experienced clinicians, and experts in research and clinical practice. Addiction is now defined as "a primary, chronic disease of brain reward, motivation, memory and related circuitry. Dysfunction in these circuits leads to characteristic biological, psychological, social, and spiritual manifestations. This is reflected in an individual pathologically pursuing reward and/or relief by substance use and other behaviours."

Increasing awareness and understanding of addictive thinking, feeling, and behaviour is critical for everyone affected by Addiction. These are indicators of how active the disease is and whether a person is engaging in healthy recovery. Addiction is a life-long disease, but there can be periods of relapse and remission. Being in tune with addictive thinking, feeling and behaviour is important in mitigating relapse, which is discussed in Chapters 3 through 5.

In Chapter 6, we shift from a focus on the disease to holistic recovery from a bio-psycho-social-spiritual perspective. This chapter looks at the important components of recovery including self-management and peer and professional support. We discuss goal setting and the essentials of continuing care. Lastly, we discuss post-acute withdrawal syndrome (PAWS), associated symptoms, and how long they can persist.

Chapter 7 is geared towards family members, highlighting that the effects of active Addiction extend well beyond the individual. Addiction is a family disease and everyone in the family plays a role in sustaining recovery. Healthy boundaries, communication, self-care, and emotional healing are discussed in more detail to help family members live a balanced and healthy life.

Chapter 8 is for health care providers who want to learn more about the importance of assessment and tailored treatment, rather than the common, current view of trying to match a patient to a packaged program. This chapter provides details regarding current issues in assessment, various treatment modalities, and barriers to treatment. It also explores the importance of education and training for health care professionals and the use of individualized treatment plans.

The title of the book, *Addiction is Addiction*, was chosen to highlight the many facets of the disease. Whether a person's drug problem involves alcohol, heroin, or prescription medication, or they engage in compulsive behaviours involving gambling, sex, relationships, or food, these are not mutually exclusive and represent different manifestations of the same disease. Many people still focus on substance use, believing that the specific behaviour is the problem. If it is simply stopped or controlled, the person will go back to being normal and this equates to health. When Addiction is present, this is not the case.

It is critical to understand what is happening in the brain because it is involved in everything we do, including how we think, feel, behave, and get along with others. The brain is the organ of judgment, personality, character, and decision-making. When your brain works properly, you work properly. When your brain is troubled, you are much more likely to be troubled and malfunction, without necessarily being aware of it.[1]

Throughout the book, we have capitalized Addiction rather than writing 'addiction' to emphasize that it is a proper noun and the name of a serious disease. It is not to be taken lightly, as it can cause disability or premature death, especially when left untreated or treated inadequately. We believe that using the lower case would perpetuate the misunderstandings related to this disease, and our goal is to shake up people's conception with the hope that their beliefs will come into alignment with the scientific evidence and reality of people living with this disease.

As with other chronic diseases, there are variable manifestations in severity that require people affected to take on self-care responsibilities. The disease is not anybody's fault, but individual responsibility is needed for recovery. This needs to be done in the context of support from family members, friends, the community, and health care providers.

We have also used case studies and examples in the book that come from our daily work with people living with Addiction and working on recovery. These are composites, meaning that we have combined different people's stories into one. We thank every one of the people we have seen over the years, as it is through all of them that we learn more about this disease every day.

The intent of this book is to encourage more open and honest dialogue about Addiction. We appreciate that there are different viewpoints and some will not agree with ours, but our hope is to cultivate an attitude of curiosity, open mindedness, and empathy. We have included appendices with additional information as well as some tools to be used in recovery, as well as a glossary of terms to explain the concepts and definitions of words used within this book.

If you are questioning whether you or someone you know may have Addiction, the following self-test addresses well-known markers or red flags for the disease.

ADDICTION SELF-TEST

1. Have you felt annoyed by others criticizing your drinking, drug use, or problem behaviour (e.g., food, sex, gambling, video games, work, exercise, etc.)?

2. Have you felt bad or guilty about your drinking, drug use, or problem behaviour?

3. Have you had to drink, use drugs or engage in problem behaviour first thing in the morning to steady your nerves or get rid of physical symptoms of discomfort, such as a headache?

4. Have you felt that you should cut down on your drinking, drug use, or problem behaviour?

5. Have you ever used drinking, drug use, or problem behaviour to numb your feelings or as an 'escape'?

6. Have you ever felt a loss of control over your drinking, drug use, or problem behaviour and used more or for longer than intended?

7. Have you had unmanageability in your life as a result of your drinking, drug use, or problem behaviour (e.g., problems at work, home, with money, or feeling stressed and overwhelmed)?

8. Have you had difficulty abstaining from drinking, drug use, or problem behaviour for extended periods?

9. Have you made promises to yourself or loved ones about quitting drinking, drug use, or other problem behaviours and then broken them?

10. Have you sought treatment in the past for drinking, drug use, or problem behaviour?

11. Do you struggle to identify, process, or communicate your feelings with yourself or others?

12. Do you find yourself over- or under-reacting emotionally to situations?

If you answered 'yes' to one or more of these questions, you may benefit from consulting with a professional to explore these challenges as you are at risk for having the disease of Addiction, if it has not already manifested in your life.

Chapter 1: Understanding Addiction

In this chapter, we focus on the biology of Addiction. We discuss how behaviour is controlled by the brain and why Addiction is considered a disease. We also cover the relationship between Addiction, mental health problems, psychiatric disorders, and trauma.

THE BRAIN AND BEHAVIOUR

All behaviour is the result of brain function, which correlates with perception, memory, motivation, learning, and action. The brain is the most complex organ in the human body and remains the least understood. What we commonly call the mind is a manifestation of a set of operations carried out by the brain. Its actions underlie not only simple motor behaviours such as walking or eating, but also all the complex cognitive actions such as thoughts, feelings, and perceptions. All the behavioural disorders that characterize psychiatric illness are disturbances of brain function. These can manifest as disorders of affect (feeling) or cognition (thinking). Neuroscientific brain research[1] and brain imaging have given us a clearer picture of how specific parts of the brain operate, and their relationship to the brain's other activities.

Problem behaviours arise when one part of the brain is under- or over-functioning. This can produce common symptoms such as irritability, impulsivity, compulsivity, obsession, hyperactivity, anxiety, and depression. The signs and symptoms can manifest in behavioural problems as well, which can lead to a psychiatric diagnosis and medication(s). This may mask or suppress the symptoms, but may not necessarily address the root problem in brain function that goes beyond the correction of a hypothetical chemical imbalance.

In Addiction, behaviours are not the disease, nor do they cause it. Behaviours are a manifestation of brain function, which are a consequence of increased or decreased activity in specific regions of the brain. This can suggest impairment in brain function due to genetic predisposition and further damage resulting from the use of alcohol and other drugs. This perspective on brain function focuses on the biological part of the problem and hopefully will allow people to get away from the stigma and shame that somehow it is the individual's fault in making bad choices, resulting in bad behaviour. In fact, one must appreciate that, since the brain is what one uses to make sense of whatever is happening within and around us, people would not know if or when the brain is providing misinformation due to some dysfunction. In other words, it is impossible to be objective about how our own brain is functioning and be fully aware of how our behaviours appear to others.

Areas of the brain impacted by Addiction that affect behaviour include the limbic system and the pre-frontal cortex.[2] They are located in the front part of the brain and set the emotional tone of the mind through the filtering of old memories, called emotional colouring, and tag new information and events as important or not, based on our past experiences. The limbic system regulates our motivation, appetite and sleep cycles, attachment and bonding, sex drive, and directly processes the sense of smell. Hence, when there are problems in the limbic system related to Addiction, the person may display moodiness, irritability, negative perceptions, emotional instability, and social isolation in addition to appetite, sleep, and sexual problems. The pre-frontal cortex regulates our attention span, judgment, impulse control, organization, learning from past experience, and ability to have feelings, especially empathy. Pre-frontal cortex dysfunction creates short attention span, easy distractibility, poor time management, unavailability of feelings, poor judgment, memory problems, social anxiety, and difficulty learning from experience.

The limbic system and pre-frontal cortex are intimately connected to the hypothalamus, which is the key location of the reward circuitry, the core of which is the connections between the ventral tegmental area (VTA) and nucleus accumbens (NA). The reward circuit is driven by healthy releases of dopamine, a brain neurotransmitter, when all is well. If the circuit has problems, reward seeking is triggered through the use of substances and other behaviours. This becomes more dysfunctional when driven by alcohol and other drugs, or addictive behaviours such as eating, sexual acting out, or gambling.

In fact, the common feature in all aspects of Addiction is the desire to escape reality through wanting more, even of necessary behaviours such as sleep, shopping, exercise, or work. This happens when reality feels overwhelming and does not match the fantasy created by the brain. This fantasy is generated by dysfunction in brain circuits related to reward, motivation, and memory.[3] It is unclear whether there is a deficiency in dopamine release, sometimes called 'low dopamine tone', or if there are problems in feedback mechanisms where the dopamine release is curtailed in the face of massive release due to the use of addictive substances and engagement in addictive behaviours. There is the well-known phenomenon of anhedonia in withdrawal, where activities that would be normally pleasurable or rewarding are no longer desirable. This has led to some speculation about the response to dopamine being blunted, the dopamine receptor density being reduced, or there may be enhanced breakdown of dopamine in the reward circuitry.[4]

In a healthy brain, the cingulate gyrus allows for thinking flexibility, adaptability, cooperation, shifting attention, and ability to see various options to help one go with the flow. Therefore, dysfunction in this area leads to getting stuck on thoughts, which is obsession; getting stuck in behaviours, which is compulsion; excessive worrying or rumination; narrowing of perceptions; an over focus on physical or emotional pain rather than focusing on what is possible; and inflexibility in being able to explore options to move forward in life. These problems are part of Addiction, so the behaviours related to being oppositional, argumentative, angry, and numb happen repeatedly and unpredictably.

Brain healing requires a daily awareness of what is 'me' and what is 'not me'. In other words, the disease relates to behaviours that occur both in wellness and illness. This provides the opportunity for the healthy circuits of the brain to be reinforced and the dysfunctional circuits to lose their dominance. It is also important to remember that the dysfunctional circuits can be easily reactivated or reinforced if addictive thinking, feelings, and dysfunctional behaviours are not kept in check on an ongoing basis. This is what makes Addiction relapsing, disabling, and fatal if not recognized and treated properly.

Science has not yet clarified the extent to which diminished frontal lobe function in people with Addiction is acquired during the development of the addictive process, or how much is a pre-existing variable from genetic inheritance that contributes to the appearance and progression of the addictive process. It is clear, though, that Addiction is about the brain and how interactions among reward, motivation, memory, and various frontal lobe circuits become translated into amplified 'go' responses and diminished 'don't go' responses. Thus, Addiction is not just about the substances or behaviours that become pathologically pursued in those individuals who manifest Addiction. The 'go' is rationalized at times as a better choice than 'don't go', even though it may neither be a choice, because of the compulsion involved, nor be rational, as viewed by a professional or a loved one who knows about the previous history of behaviours under similar circumstances. This is also sometimes called a problem with incentive salience (motivation) and executive functioning (the ability to modulate impulses and compulsions in a healthy manner).

Tolerance and withdrawal are physiological adaptations caused by the brain adjusting itself to the periodic or regular presence of a chemical or substances over time, which are potentially disrupting the internal balance. We commonly hear, 'I don't have any withdrawal symptoms so I must not be addicted,' or, 'I'm addicted because I need more and more and have withdrawal if I don't get enough.' Both of these statements are misleading, as tolerance and withdrawal commonly occur with Addiction, but are not critical components in its diagnosis. Both tolerance and withdrawal occur in response to most chemicals that affect the brain, whether they produce Addiction or not.

Tolerance occurs when the brain is exposed to a chemical or substance over time, causing it to become less sensitive to a particular amount or dose, and requiring more to have the same effect. This happens because the body and brain constantly try to maintain homeostasis or balance by generating a response that is opposite of the response resulting from a substance or addictive behaviour. This is why withdrawal from alcohol, a drug that slows down many key processes in the body, involves the speeding up of these processes as the body tries to re-establish homeostasis.

Withdrawal symptoms can occur when the blood level of a particular substance is falling. This can happen in the presence or absence of the substance in the body. Even the anticipation of the use of an addictive substance or problem behaviour, which is sometimes called craving, can produce withdrawal symptoms. As Addiction is a complex, lifelong disease of the entire self beyond one's physiology, it is important to look beyond tolerance and withdrawal as sole criteria. It is also important to appreciate that the withdrawal response is stored in memory and can be triggered by people, places, and things, which can lead one to relapse. For example, going on an annual golf trip with friends which had historically included alcohol and cocaine is likely to trigger craving, may precipitate withdrawal symptoms and, thus, can lead to relapse involving drinking alcohol and/or using cocaine.

WHAT MAKES ADDICTION A DISEASE?

The term disease broadly refers to an abnormal condition that affects one or more organs in the body, which is the brain in the case of Addiction. Having a disease impairs normal function of the organ(s) involved and is therefore associated with dysfunction and disturbance of homeostasis. In other words, in Addiction the brain is not functioning properly and leads to a disruption of balance. A disease is also characterized by specific signs and symptoms that are the same in people who have the disease regardless of socio-cultural variables such as ethnicity or socio-economic status. A disease may be caused by factors originally from an external source, such as infectious disease, or by internal dysfunction, such as in diabetes. In humans, the term 'disease' is often used to refer to any condition that causes pain, dysfunction, distress, social problems, or death to the person afflicted, or similar problems for those in contact with the person. In this broader sense, it sometimes includes injuries, disabilities, disorders, syndromes, infections, isolated symptoms, deviant behaviours, and atypical variations of structure and function. Diseases not only affect people physically, but also emotionally, mentally, and spiritually, as living with many diseases can alter one's perspective on life and thus affect thinking, feeling and behaviour. The outcome of a disease may be recovery, disability, or death.

Most commonly, people equate the term disease to infectious diseases, which are clinically evident diseases that result from the presence of pathogenic microbial agents, such as viruses and bacteria. They are usually acute and time-limited in nature with or without treatment, leading to premature death or recovery. Non-infectious diseases are often chronic and last for a life time. Examples of these include most forms of cancer, heart disease, and genetic diseases, such as cystic fibrosis or sickle-cell disease. By definition, a chronic disease is one that lasts for more than six months or occurs over a life time. It may be constantly present, or it may go into remission and periodically flare-up as a relapse. A chronic disease may be stable, meaning that it does not get any worse, or it may be progressive, meaning that it gets worse over time. Most chronic diseases can be beneficially treated, even if they cannot be permanently cured. An example of a chronic infectious disease is the herpes virus, which can flare-up periodically over the lifetime of someone who is an infected carrier. Stress is commonly associated with flare-ups of this disease, which is also true of Addiction.

The present health care system in western society has emerged in response to acute diseases and injuries. An acute disease is often imposed on a person from an external source, lasts for a short time, can begin rapidly, and may have intense symptoms. Treatment for acute diseases is focused on removing the disease or shortening its course and reducing/alleviating unpleasant or painful symptoms. Treatment is typically short term with the aim of returning the person to normal as quickly as possible.

As the prevalence of chronic disease has risen over the past fifty years, acute care practices have proved increasingly inefficient and ineffective, as chronic diseases cannot be effectively treated using the same approach. With a chronic disease, the person's life is irreversibly changed and quick fixes are often not possible or realistic. At times, quick fixes can be harmful as symptoms are masked while the disease progresses. The goal in treating chronic disease is not necessarily to cure it, but maintenance of the highest possible quality of life with focus on independent living and joy, and providing assistance where needed.

Even in the presence of a chronic disease, our society remains focused on fast results and quick improvements for unpleasant or painful symptoms. Efforts can become more focused on alleviating these symptoms than understanding why they occurred in the first place. This perpetuates the Band-Aid effect. This means providing a temporary solution to a long-term problem, or something that seems to be a solution but has no real lasting, beneficial effect. Rather than face a problem, it gets covered up, such as prescribing medication to treat anxiety rather than taking a more holistic approach to address the root problems driving that fear and anxiety. Symptom management is part of the treatment plan for Addiction, but it is also necessary to have a holistic perspective rather than seeing the patient as a set of symptoms or behaviours that need to be alleviated. For example, we have had patients come to us who are struggling with symptoms of anxiety, depression, anger, drug use, relationship issues, physical pain and obsessive compulsive tendencies. They have sometimes been involved in treatment for years, focusing on each specific symptom in isolation, with little overall benefit. Understanding the larger scope of Addiction and what is happening in their brain and being allows them to simplify their treatment plan and activities, which in turns results in more definitive progress in recovery.

Many people who struggle with looking at Addiction as a disease will talk about making poor choices. Some believe that in viewing Addiction as a disease, it abdicates all responsibility for behaviour. People often become adamant that sufferers need to take responsibility for their behaviour, make restitution and learn from their mistakes to ensure that the behaviours never happen again. All human beings need to take responsibility for their behaviours and be accountable for their actions, but blaming one's self or someone else for a condition that is beyond their control only increases shame. Shame is toxic and can keep a person in active Addiction, as they stay stuck in believing it is futile to change their ways because they do not have the capacity to change and/or no one will ever trust them again anyway. When the focus shifts and the person recognizes that they did not choose to behave badly and that their behaviours are secondary to dysfunction in the brain, they can then start to focus on recovery and appreciate that the disease is only a part of them and not defining of them. A phrase that needs to be heard in recovery is: *You did not choose to get this disease, but now that you know you have it, you need to choose to focus on recovery.* Family and friends need to understand that support is needed to help in initiating and maintaining changes in recovery, such as by driving their loved one to meetings, talking about feelings, and looking at their own vulnerabilities rather than shaming, demanding, or policing them, which are various ways of controlling that do not generally work long-term.

We can further examine the disease analogy using diabetes as a comparison. Diabetes[5] is a group of metabolic problems that are chronic in nature. With type 1 diabetes, it is believed that a combination of genetic predisposition and additional, as yet unidentified, factors provoke the immune system into attacking and killing the insulin-producing cells in the pancreas. Type 2 diabetes is mainly caused by insulin resistance in the cells. This means that no matter how much or how little insulin is made, the body cannot use it as well as it needs to. Over time, the excess sugar in the blood gradually poisons the pancreas, causing it to make less insulin and making it even more difficult to keep blood glucose under control. High blood sugar causes damage to the vasculature, which interferes with blood circulation in various areas of the body such as heart and brain, leading to more complications.

Lifestyle choices such as poor eating habits and lack of exercise increase a person's vulnerability to diabetes. Currently, obesity is a leading cause of developing insulin resistance and approximately 80% of people with type 2 diabetes are overweight. Some can argue that people's lifestyle choices cause them to get diabetes, but the majority of society now accepts that diabetes is a chronic disease with a multitude of risk factors, and that lifestyle choices increase one's vulnerability. Once a person has been diagnosed with diabetes, it is prudent for them to make healthier lifestyle choices. However, once they have it, they cannot go back to not having the disease. Further, the poor lifestyle choices implicated in diabetes may be related to Addiction involving food in an individual, so diabetes is, at times, a complication of Addiction. Just like diabetes, Addiction also causes complications in various organs, depending on what drugs and behaviours may be part of a person's Addiction.

With Addiction, some people have difficulty accepting that it is chronic in nature and want to put it behind them. Health care providers and family members can perpetuate this belief by hoping and expecting a cure. However, this viewpoint is a set-up for the person affected for relapse or the continued progression of the disease, particularly if they have not made the necessary changes in their life to maintain healthy recovery on a consistent basis. It can also lead to lying and minimizing or hiding the symptoms that require attention. Without treatment or engagement in recovery activities, Addiction is progressive and can result in disability or premature death.

ADDICTION AS A PRIMARY, CHRONIC BRAIN DISEASE

Addiction is a primary, chronic disease of brain reward, motivation, memory, and related circuitry as defined by the American Society of Addiction Medicine (ASAM). Primary means that it is not caused by anything else and chronic means that it is lifelong in nature. Once someone has the disease of Addiction, it does not go away. A common question asked in treatment is, 'what caused me to become addicted?' Often, people want to look for the cause of their substance use or addictive behaviour and have difficulty understanding that there are many risk factors, aggravating factors, and vulnerabilities, but nothing causes it necessarily, as research has pointed to genetics as the fundamental contributor. This is similar to cancer, for which we know many risk factors that can be addressed, yet someone can still get cancer without them, or not get cancer despite having risk factors such as being a smoker for many years. Addiction works the same way; a person can have many risk factors but not develop the disease, whereas someone who does not have many risk factors may develop it. Addiction is considered a primary disease even more so because trying to treat a perceived cause, such as trauma, can actually worsen it if adequate treatment and support is not provided for recovery.

Addiction is about differences in brain functioning of people with the disease, not about their use of specific substances such as alcohol, cocaine, or nicotine, or problems related to behaviours like excessive eating, exercising, or gambling. This paradigm clearly describes Addiction as a discrete condition, separate from substance-related or behavioural problems, and the problems are recognized as consequences of the disease. The definition from ASAM describes Addiction as a single condition—Addiction is Addiction—rather than describing 'addictions' such as that involving alcohol as distinct from Addiction involving cocaine or gambling. This is a contrast to other classification systems, in which each substance- or behaviour-related problem is considered to be separate.

The decision to have the first sentence of the ASAM definition clearly specify the involvement of memory, motivation, and related circuitry was made to reinforce the idea of Addiction as a brain disease with a biological basis, with behaviour being a manifestation rather than the cause. It is also recognized that Addiction is not just a brain disease. Beyond the biological aspect, disease manifestations occur along psychological, social, and spiritual dimensions. A number of people look at the spiritual dimension as part of psychological or social, but spirituality is fundamentally about the basic values a person has and what gives meaning to a person's life. Values and meaning in life provide a framework for a human being's relationship to themselves, with others and with the transcendent aspect of life or existential connection with the rest of the universe.

Most researchers state unequivocally that heredity is a critical factor in developing Addiction and an individual has a 25% or greater risk if one parent has the disease. This risk obviously increases if both parents have the disease, as the individual inherits the genes from both parents. Addiction has been classified as genetically complex, meaning there are many genes that play a role in shaping it. This may account for its many manifestations and individual subtleties.

Genetic factors[6] alone account for approximately 50-60% of the likelihood that an individual will develop Addiction. However, having a genetic predisposition does not guarantee that Addiction will occur because environment also plays a significant role. Over the past twenty years, a new area of science called epigenetics has influenced how professionals view Addiction and many other diseases, and has broadened our understanding of the roles of nature and nurture. At its most basic level, epigenetics[7] is the study of changes in gene activity and how the genome responds to the environment. Stress, exposure to substances, family, culture, and other factors activate chemical switches that regulate how the Addiction genes are expressed. In order for genes to express themselves or be 'switched on', environmental factors need to interact with the person's biology, which then affects the extent to which the genetic factors exert their influence.

There is likely no uncontaminated gene pool for Addiction, and all humans are vulnerable. We live in a world that fosters instant gratification, the desire for more, and easy access to mood- altering and socially acceptable substances such as alcohol. With the Internet and changing technology, gambling, video games, and pornography are more accessible to individuals of all ages, including children. Resiliencies an individual does or does not acquire through family and culture can affect the extent to which genetic predispositions lead to behavioural and other manifestations of Addiction. These factors influence self-concept and behaviour, as well as how people interact with others, react to stress, and deal with feelings in healthy or unhealthy ways.

Factors that can contribute to the appearance of Addiction, leading to its characteristic bio-psycho-socio-spiritual manifestations, as outlined in the ASAM definition include:

a. The presence of an underlying biological deficit in the function of reward circuits, such that drugs and behaviours that enhance reward function are preferred and sought as reinforcers;

b. Repeated engagement in drug use or other addictive behaviours, causing neuroadaptation in motivational circuitry and leading to impaired control over further drug use or engagement in addictive behaviours;

c. Cognitive and affective distortions, which impair perceptions and compromise the ability to deal with feelings, resulting in significant self-deception;

d. Disruption of healthy social supports and problems in interpersonal relationships that impact the development or impact of resiliencies;

e. Exposure to trauma or stressors that overwhelm an individual's coping abilities;

f. Distortion in meaning, purpose, and values that guide attitudes, thinking, and behaviour;

g. Distortions in a person's connection with self, with others and with the transcendent (referred to as God by many, the Higher Power by 12-steps groups, or higher consciousness by others); and

h. The presence of co-occurring psychiatric disorders in persons who engage in substance use or other addictive behaviours.

Addiction is characterized by:

A. Inability to consistently **A**bstain,

B. Impairment in **B**ehavioural control,

C. **C**raving or increased hunger for drugs or rewarding experiences,

D. **D**iminished recognition of significant problems with one's behaviours and interpersonal relationships, and

E. A dysfunctional **E**motional response

Addiction affects neurotransmission and interactions within reward structures of the brain, including the nucleus accumbens, anterior cingulate cortex, basal forebrain, and amygdala, such that motivational hierarchies are altered and addictive behaviours are reinforced. This may or may not include alcohol and other drug use, and supplant healthy, self-care related behaviours. Addiction also affects neurotransmission and interactions between cortical and hippocampal circuits connected to brain reward structures, such that the memory of previous exposures to rewards such as food, sex, alcohol, and other drugs, lead to a biological and behavioural response to external cues, in turn triggering craving or engagement in addictive behaviours.

The neurobiology of Addiction encompasses more than the neurochemistry of reward. The frontal cortex of the brain and underlying white matter connections between the frontal cortex and circuits of reward, motivation, and memory are fundamental in the manifestations of altered impulse control, altered judgment, and the dysfunctional pursuit of rewards despite consequences seen in Addiction. Often the affected person expresses a desire to be 'normal', despite cumulative adverse consequences experienced from engagement in substance use and other addictive behaviours. The frontal lobes are important in inhibiting impulsivity and in assisting individuals to appropriately delay gratification. When individuals with Addiction have problems deferring gratification, there is a neurological basis for it in the frontal cortex, representing a deficit in executive functioning. Frontal lobe morphology, connectivity, and functioning are still in the process of maturation during adolescence and young adulthood, and early exposure to substance use is another significant factor in the development of Addiction. Many neuroscientists believe that developmental morphology is the basis that makes early-life exposure to substances such an important factor.

Addiction is more than a behavioural disorder. It affects a person's behaviour, thinking, feelings, and interactions with others, including their ability to relate to members of their family, community, their own psychological state, and events that occur in their daily experience.

Cognitive changes in Addiction can include:

a. Preoccupation with substance use;

b. Altered evaluations of the relative benefits and detriments associated with drugs or rewarding behaviours; and

c. The inaccurate belief that problems experienced in one's life are attributable to other causes rather than being a predictable consequence of Addiction.

The persistent risk or recurrences of relapse after periods of abstinence are another fundamental feature of Addiction. This can be triggered by exposure to rewarding substances and behaviours, environmental cues to use, and emotional stressors that trigger heightened activity in brain stress circuits. In the 12-step program, people, places, and things are referred to as powerful triggers for relapse. This is because the memory circuitry is activated by each of these. Individuals in treatment have shared how the smell of wine, the taste of non-alcoholic beer, the sound of slot machines, the sight of fast food commercials on TV, or a caressing touch from the opposite sex can all elicit intense memories and feelings that can trigger relapse. Typically, the individual is unaware and needs someone external to them (i.e., peer support, therapist, sponsor) to identify the risks and triggers.

Clinical interventions can be quite effective in altering the course of Addiction. Close monitoring of behaviours and contingency management can contribute to positive clinical outcomes. Contingency management is where tangible rewards are given to reinforce healthy behaviour. For instance, giving medallions and having celebrations in 12-step meetings to reinforce milestones of abstinence. This can also sometimes include behavioural consequences for relapse behaviours, such as a parent taking away financial support for their adult child who are not making a clear commitment to recovery. Engagement in health promotion activities that promote personal responsibility and accountability, connection with others, and personal growth also contribute to recovery. We explore these health promotion activities throughout the book, and particular in the holistic recovery chapter.

The qualitative ways in which the brain and behaviour respond to drug exposure and engagement in addictive behaviours are different at later stages of Addiction than in earlier stages, indicating progression that may not be overtly apparent to the individual. As is the case with other chronic diseases, the condition must be monitored and managed over time to:

a. Decrease the frequency and intensity of relapses;

b. Sustain periods of remission; and

c. Optimize the person's level of functioning during periods of remission.

In some cases of Addiction, medication management can improve treatment outcomes. Typically, the integration of psycho-social-spiritual rehabilitation and ongoing care with evidence-based pharmacological therapy can be expected to provide the best results. Chronic disease management is important for minimization of episodes of relapse and their impact. Treatment of Addiction saves lives.

It is important to view relapse as a process in which the physical event of using is the culmination or manifestation of earlier signs and symptoms. The physical part may include craving or post-acute withdrawal symptoms. They are usually preceded by persistent thinking distortions and emotional lability, which is preceded by loss of or diminished spiritual connections.

Relapse after a period of abstinence can result in death due to an overdose if the person has lost his or her tolerance, such that the dose of the drug that was not a problem before can become fatal.

ADDICTION, MENTAL HEALTH, AND PSYCHIATRIC DISORDERS

Mental health problems are common and occur in all of us. We all feel sad, mad, or bad from time to time. People have different coping styles based on our experience and environment to deal with whatever is going on that is unpleasant or unpalatable. Addiction as a brain disease creates a vulnerability in which mental health problems are either ignored, avoided, or magnified, especially in terms of blaming other people, places, or things rather than taking personal responsibility. Feelings are often repressed and suppressed, meaning that they are either unconsciously or purposefully forgotten or minimized. When this occurs, the feelings commonly come out in the form of anxiety and depression as one can only ignore them for so long.

Anxiety related problems are fear-based. The fear is usually of things in the future that may or may not happen, yet the person experiences them as if they were happening right then, thus creating an overwhelming emotional response that the individual wants to escape from. Fear and anxiety are common when someone with Addiction does not know how or when they will get their next hit of a drug, in addition to anxiety being a common withdrawal reaction that physiologically results in more drug seeking. Panic attacks are an extreme example that can happen in the context of substance/ behaviour use or withdrawal. A panic attack indicates that there are many feelings that have been ignored and need to be processed.

Depression is also a common withdrawal symptom connected to all aspects of Addiction, both chemical and behavioural. It is a reflection of the distress experienced when one cannot get what one desires, is losing what one desires, or realizes that what was once pleasurable is no longer. It reflects the increasing recognition that one is at a place where one did not want to be. Depression is usually associated with regret, guilt, and shame, which in thinking escalates from 'I shouldn't have done that' to 'I did bad' to 'I am bad.' The chemical imbalance that results in the brain related to depression may require anti-depressant treatment; however, these medications are usually ineffective if one remains in active Addiction, with or without ongoing alcohol or drug use. Further, the long-term utility of anti-depressant medications remains dubious.

Prolonged problems with anxiety and depression, together with problems in behaviour, can result in more entrenched diagnoses of psychiatric disorders such as generalized anxiety disorder, depressive disorder, or bipolar disorder. It is essential to look closely because the prognosis is much better if these are a complication of Addiction because the symptoms that led to these diagnoses often remit once Addiction is treated effectively and the individual maintains ongoing recovery. This is done by assessing for Addiction using the ABCDE characteristics mentioned earlier as well as understanding how people approach relationships and what drives their motivation to engage in behaviours, including substance use.

Psychiatric diagnoses such as attention deficit disorder (ADD), attention deficit hyperactivity disorder (ADHD), and borderline personality disorder (BPD) are also part of Addiction, rather than separate entities as they are made out to be by some professionals. More severe mental illness, such as schizophrenia or psychoses, can occur concurrently with Addiction, thus requiring more intensive and specialized treatment with medication. In these situations, proper medications, close monitoring, and continuing care are critical to maintaining healthy recovery.

TRAUMA

Human brain function is dependent on the physical, chemical, and emotional environment, such that it can go into dysfunction acutely or chronically when exposed to trauma. This can include physical trauma like brain injury, chemical trauma like exposure to substances, and emotional trauma like physical, emotional, or sexual abuse. The vulnerability is greatest during fetal development in pregnancy and early childhood development, from birth to age six as the brain undergoes a significant amount of growth and change during early childhood. Age seven to sixteen is a period of rapid learning and development that includes development of healthy self-concept and interpersonal relationships. This can be hampered by trauma which can generate fear, anger, and shame that may or may not be articulated clearly; and result in behavioural problems. Between the ages of seventeen and twenty-five, executive functioning, decision-making, and becoming responsible adults can become compromised if exposure to trauma occurs. Risk-taking behaviours like speeding, certain sports, and not following safety protocol that are common during late adolescence and early adult life are part of growing up, yet create a vulnerability to all forms of trauma, and can hamper further development.

Some people erroneously believe that trauma is the cause of Addiction. As mentioned already, Addiction is a primary disease meaning that it cannot be spontaneously caused by anything, as it usually already exists in the genetics of the beholder. The reality is that not everyone who experiences trauma goes on to suffer from Addiction and many people with Addiction have had no trauma prior to the disease manifesting. Adverse childhood events (ACE) that are associated with a lot of negative health outcomes during adulthood, including Addiction, are aggravating factors, not causes. As trauma is a strong aggravating factor in Addiction, it must be dealt with in the framework of recovery, meaning that the emotional repercussions of the trauma need to be addressed, but only when there is a recovery framework in place and some stability in recovery is established. Dealing directly with the trauma in therapy without that leads to more emotional pain, thus increasing the desire to escape, which makes Addiction worse, which heightens the emotional pain from the trauma, thus keeping people trapped in suffering and despair. It is the genetic predisposition, combined with a host of environmental issues, including but not limited to trauma, that determines when and how the disease of Addiction becomes visible.

Post-traumatic stress disorder (PTSD) is a specific psychiatric disorder that is often present in people with Addiction, and can also be present without. When one appreciates the brain vulnerability, it is easy to understand that someone who has manifest Addiction or a high degree of genetic predisposition would be more prone to PTSD. The inability to deal with feelings in a healthy manner creates conditions in the brain in which repeated flashbacks occur of emotionally charged situations that were overwhelming and/or confusing. Intrusive memories represent interference by the past with present brain function and can lead to erratic behaviour, aggression, nightmares, and sleep dysfunction. Commonly prescribed pain or anti-anxiety medications that may provide initial quick relief ultimately make addiction-related problems worse. These medications may aggravate the condition at the level of the brain as well as promote suppression of feelings, which build up and drive the disease further. Treating PTSD as a separate entity does not make Addiction go away. Rather, treating Addiction makes PTSD treatment more effective, largely because there is considerable overlap between the effective treatment approaches, such as individual and group psychotherapy for dealing with painful memories and feelings.

CHAPTER SUMMARY

All behaviour is the result of brain function. With Addiction, behaviours are not the disease, nor do they cause it. When viewing behaviour as a manifestation of brain function, it is evident that problem behaviours are the symptoms of abnormal functioning in the brain. The ability to make healthy choices is lost in Addiction and behaviours can aggravate the disease or help lead to recovery. The term 'disease' broadly refers to a dysfunctional state or an abnormal condition that affects one or more organs. The brain is the organ that is impacted in Addiction. Having a disease impairs normal function of the organ(s) involved and is therefore associated with disruption of normal homeostasis or balance. It is characterized by specific signs and symptoms that become increasingly dysfunctional and problematic. Appreciating Addiction as a primary, chronic brain disease requires an understanding of the terms. Primary means that it is not caused by anything else, and chronic means that it is lifelong in its myriad manifestations.

Mental health problems are common and occur in all of us. Addiction, however, creates vulnerabilities such that mental health problems are ignored, avoided, or magnified. Feelings are often repressed or suppressed such that they commonly come out in the form of anxiety and depression. Treating them as separate diagnoses without addressing Addiction can be problematic. Trauma is not the cause of Addiction but it is definitely a strong aggravating factor and must be dealt with in the framework of recovery. Some stability is needed with recovery structure, as trauma therapy without that leads to more emotional pain, thus increasing the desire to escape, which makes Addiction worse. If Addiction is left untreated, it will result in institutionalization or premature death. However, there is tremendous hope within the treatment of Addiction for a high quality of life.

Chapter 2: Historical Perspectives and the Birth of the Definition of Addiction

In this chapter, we trace the history of Addiction from the eighteenth to the twenty-first century, and discuss the short version of the definition of Addiction as currently accepted by medical specialists. We also explore the characteristics of Addiction in depth using case examples.

The word Addiction has not been widely used as a medical diagnosis historically and, to date, there continues to be stigma attached to it. Other terms commonly used include 'substance abuse' or 'substance dependence' or 'substance use disorder', but it has become evident that changing the terms has caused much confusion, while stigma about Addiction persists. Decades of scientific research has clearly established that Addiction is a brain disease[1] and is more complex than just the substance use or addictive behaviour. Addiction as a disease has not been a widely accepted viewpoint and lack of knowledge and understanding persists, even amongst professionals. Many professionals continue to put emphasis on Addiction as bad behaviour, poor choices, moral failing, or weakness, with little or no understanding of what is happening in the brain that is driving behaviour. Many of the common misconceptions that Addiction is about these or other things, like self-medication, selfishness, or enjoyment does not fit with what is known and understood about the disease.

Addiction is a primary, chronic disease of brain dysfunction and is about pathologically seeking reward and/or relief, as we discussed in Chapter 1. It also involves memory distortion, neglecting self, motivation problems, and impaired behavioural control. Distortions in thinking, feeling, and perceptions are part of the disease, while the behaviours people see are a manifestation of it. They are not the disease, nor are they its cause. The persistence of these behaviours reinforces the disease and sadly, focusing only on changing behaviours and controlling symptoms can create more resistance for the disease, as it is not sufficient to deal with Addiction. For instance, attempts to stop obsessive-compulsive tendencies with cleaning often leads to greater discomfort, such that the person uses alcohol to then manage that discomfort. What can also happen are that attempts to control drinking lead to discomfort that drives acting out with overeating fast food. Focusing on symptom management alone allows Addiction to thrive and may force it to find a new home.

FROM THE EIGHTEENTH TO THE TWENTY-FIRST CENTURY

The term 'alcoholic disease syndrome' was used by a prominent American, Dr. Benjamin Rush,[2] back in 1784. In the nineteenth century, 'inebriety'[3] was recognized by some as a disease, which manifested as alcoholism and drug addiction. Another term frequently used to refer to alcoholism towards the end of the nineteenth century was 'dipsomania'. Both of these terms referred to the behaviours of excessive drinking and intoxication. Dr. Jellinek, an American physician who began to study alcoholism and its complications, most notably liver cirrhosis in the 1940s, further explored the concept of alcoholism as a disease and referred to 'alcohol addiction' for almost two decades prior to the publication of his best known work, *The Disease Concept of Alcoholism* (1960). He also described phases of Addiction involving alcohol in an attempt to capture the diversity of how the disease manifested. It is important to appreciate that the focus seemed to be on intoxication and people today still struggle with knowing when intoxication is acceptable and when is it a problem. Many strive to control the problem by trying to avoid intoxication, yet it is a hard lesson for individuals, families, and society to learn that the disease is far bigger than the problems related to being drunk.

The establishment of Alcoholics Anonymous[4] in the 1930s led to more discussion of alcoholism as a disease characterized by loss of control over alcohol use and over one's life. It was described in *The Big Book* (1939) as an "obsession of the mind" (p. 23) and a "physical allergy of the body" (p. xxviii). The combination of the allergy and obsession contribute to the powerlessness and unmanageability that are part of step 1 of Alcoholics Anonymous. Step 1 is, "We admitted we were powerless over alcohol... That our lives had become unmanageable." It took another twenty years for the disease concept to appear again in academic literature. It can be argued that medical authors' appreciation of a primary disease called Addiction remains spotty, as people still argue whether it is a social or moral problem.[5] In India, for example, the prevalent terminology has been "de-addiction". This focuses solely on solving the Addiction problem by stopping the behaviours, treating withdrawal, and considering the problem solved until the inevitable relapse happens, which is then called "re-addiction".

The World Health Organization (WHO) acknowledged difficulties in developing a definition of Addiction in its report in 1952.[6] The WHO struggled with terms such as "drug dependence" and "habituation" that were being used to describe drug-related harms, but provided no real direction for diagnosis or treatment based on those distinctions. "Habituation" was considered a less severe form of psychological adaptation. The separation of alcohol from other drugs has also been an issue. For example, in the 1970s, the U.S. Congress established two separate research agencies within the National Institutes of Health—the NIAAA (National Institute on Alcohol Abuse and Alcoholism) for alcohol research and NIDA (National Institute on Drug Abuse) for research on drugs.

By the 1960s, there was an increasing consensus within the WHO to drop the terms "habituation" and "addiction" in favor of "drug dependence". A 1969 WHO report called for using the term drug dependence, with tolerance and withdrawal, which are often collectively called physical dependence, becoming the only necessary conditions for its diagnosis. Similarly, the difference between diagnoses of alcohol dependence in lieu of the comparatively minor syndrome of alcohol abuse was the presence of physical dependence in the form of pharmacological tolerance, meaning needing more to feel an effect, or characteristic withdrawal symptoms. In 1978, the WHO similarly called for use of the term alcohol dependence syndrome (ADS) in lieu of the term alcoholism. Sadly, changing terms only added to the confusion.

Some concerned doctors in New York City, led by Dr. Ruth Fox, established the New York City Medical Committee on Alcoholism in 1951, which became the New York City Medical Society on Alcoholism (NYCMSA) in 1954. The American Medical Society on Alcoholism (AMSA) was the next step in 1967, which grew into the American Medical Society on Alcohol and Other Drug Dependencies (AMSAODD) in 1983 by joining with the California Society for Treatment of Alcoholism and Other Drug Dependencies (CSTAODD) that was established in 1972. Leadership by physicians such as Dr. Stan Gitlow, Dr. Sheila Blume, Dr. LeClair Bissell, Dr. Jess Bromley, Dr. Max Schneider, Dr. Doug Talbott, and Dr. David Smith helped guide the development of the field of Addiction Medicine. Through the 1980s, it was increasingly felt that Addiction was the word that needed to be clarified. Hence, AMSAODD became the American Society of Addiction Medicine (ASAM) and was accepted by the American Medical Association (AMA) as a medical specialty society in 1988. A designated code for Addiction Medicine, ADM, was approved by the AMA Board of Trustees in 1990, by which physicians could self-designate their primary area of clinical specialization. These actions by ASAM and the AMA created a need to clearly define both Addiction and Addiction Medicine.

In Canada, the Canadian Medical Society on Alcohol and Other Drugs (CMSAOD) was founded in 1988 under the leadership of Dr. Jim Rankin, and its inaugural meeting was held in Calgary in 1989. CMSAOD became the Canadian Society of Addiction Medicine (C*SAM) in 1997 under the leadership of Dr. Raju Hajela. There had been considerable work done in Canada through the 1940s onwards, especially in Ontario with the creation of Alcoholism Research Foundation (ARF) in Toronto. Dr. Gordon Bell was a pioneering physician who started to treat alcoholics in his own home in the late 1940s. Dr. Bell was often under scrutiny by his colleagues for dealing with these so-called 'degenerates.' He always treated patients with Addiction respectfully and felt that proper treatment was essential to help people achieve sobriety. He succeeded in establishing the Donwood Institute in 1967 as the premier alcoholism treatment facility in Toronto. ARF went through a few transformations over the decades to become the Alcohol and Drug Research Foundation (ADRF) and then the Addiction Research Foundation (ARF) again. ARF and the Donwood Institute were later absorbed into the current Centre for Addiction and Mental Health (CAMH), together with the Clarke Institute of Psychiatry and the Queen Street Mental Health Centre.

The idea that Addiction is an illness and needs to be understood as a brain disease was emphasized by Alan Leshner, PhD, Director of National Institute of Drug Abuse (NIDA), in 1997. He hypothesized that prolonged effects of drugs on the brain manifested as a chronic, relapsing, compulsive disease that had behavioural and social-context embedded with it. He made clear that substances of abuse had rewarding properties through their action on specific reward circuitry in the brain.

Research on reward circuitry has revealed that dopamine surges in the brain for all humans are normally driven by food and sex with a feedback mechanism of satiation, which says 'enough'. However, with psychoactive drugs and Addiction, the same circuit becomes associated with saying 'more'.[7] Repeated exposure to psychoactive drugs and their rewarding effects is one of the pathways that make the disease visible.

Genetic predisposition as the other precursor to the manifestation of the disease also came to be increasingly recognized over the last five decades. The noteworthy point is that discoveries in genetics point to Addiction as a single condition rather than Addiction involving alcohol and drugs being separate.

Clinicians grappling with substance-related problems in their patients came to commonly refer to the 3Cs, or later the 4Cs—loss of or impaired control; craving; compulsion; and continued use despite harm—as being the features of Addiction. Further challenges to understanding occurred in the diagnostic distinctions found in the Diagnostic and Statistical Manual of Mental Disorders, or DSM,[8] established as a standard by the American Psychiatric Association (APA). The DSM (1980, 1987, 1994, 2000) classified substance use disorders as either substance abuse or substance dependence on the basis of a checklist of behavioural symptoms and signs. The difference between substance abuse and substance dependence being continued use despite harm due to lack of knowledge vs. impaired control was implied but not clearly understood by all practitioners or patients. Hence, there was persistent confusion over whether Addiction was synonymous with substance dependence only or with abuse as well. Recently the DSM 5, released in 2013, eliminated the two diagnostic categories and merged them into one condition called substance use disorder, which can be mild, moderate, or severe, depending on how many of the eleven behavioural criteria are endorsed. Sadly, the APA and DSM remain silent in defining Addiction and focus on behavioural symptoms only.

In Canada, by 1999 a group of clinicians associated with the C*SAM felt that there was enough evidence available to recognize that the characteristic feature of Addiction was 'impaired control'. These words were selected over 'loss of control' to highlight that this was a gradually progressive problem once it manifested and was not a simple on/off phenomenon. One does not need to look for a complete absence of control, such as daily drinking to excess, for Addiction to be present.

The problem of Addiction involving opioids, specifically heroin, was well recognized through the twentieth century. Yet, through the 1990s, North America saw the beginnings of an emerging epidemic of misuse, diversion, and associated morbidity and mortality from prescription opioids that were used for the treatment of chronic pain. It was clear that as the prescribing of opioids expanded through that decade, many developed pharmacological tolerance or experienced withdrawal symptoms if they overused their medication and ran out early. Some labeled tolerance and withdrawal to be physical dependence and were confused as to whether that was Addiction or not, while others minimized the risk and continued the opioids for pain, without appreciation for addiction-related problems that may be emerging or persisting.

Clinicians have long recognized that brief educational interventions lead to behaviour change with substance abuse. However, with substance dependence, which is often considered synonymous with Addiction, treatment needs to occur in the chronic disease framework and brief behavioural or educational interventions are insufficient for producing change. Unfortunately, this episodic treatment model, when used for substance dependence, perpetuated the myth that once someone was taught skills in a psycho-educational treatment program, they should be able to self-manage with or without support. This confusion persists for many clinicians, especially if they label every substance-related problem as substance abuse. The interventions may be limited to cessation of use of the specific substance that was identified as the problem, such as drinking alcohol, rather than appreciating the bigger disease of Addiction that requires sustained, long- term intervention and treatment strategies.

In a clinical environment, techniques designed to help people learn new healthy behaviours and 'unlearn' problematic ones may work for those with so-called substance abuse. This is the population that these interventions were designed for, after all. At this level of problem, there are no characteristic brain changes and simpler educational and/or behavioural interventions are enough in leading to the amelioration of problem substance use or other problem behaviours. For those with substance dependence or Addiction, education is not enough and the expectation of learning new behaviours and 'unlearning' old ones quickly compounds shame and stigma by blaming the individual for not trying hard enough.

Another dimension requiring the emergence of consensus in the medical field was whether to define the disease of Addiction as a single condition, or to talk about 'addictions'—to have separate concepts for substance use disorders based on the primary substance involved, or to separate non-substance conditions from substance-related conditions. Thus, would there be the need to talk about things like alcohol addiction, opioid addiction, nicotine addiction, as well as gambling addiction, sexual addiction, video game addiction, and the like, or would there simply be Addiction? For this reason, throughout the book we refer to 'Addiction involving...' rather than specifying the type of Addiction. This is to get away from the out-of-date notion that Addiction is about what you are 'addicted to' rather than appreciating the full spectrum of thinking, feeling, spiritual and other behavioural manifestations of the disease. Referring to 'Addiction involving...' allows the patient and treatment providers to be mindful of the acute vulnerabilities that may have led to seeking help and require specific interventions, such as in 'Addiction involving opioids', though never forgetting that the disease can be manifesting in more subtle ways in other areas that require exploration in the context of chronic disease treatment.

Historically, diagnostic systems such as the DSM and International Classification of Diseases (ICD) have listed substance use disorders separately as alcohol dependence, opioid dependence, pathological gambling, etc. These distinctions have led to differences in ideology, practice, and funding for services. Consensus emerged that effective clinical interventions require that treatment address all aspects of Addiction as they are unmasked during the process of assessment, treatment, and recovery in the framework of chronic disease management and the need for continuing care. Both neuroscience and clinical experience suggest that no matter what may be the entry point of 'addicted to' for a given person, assessment and treatment need to be more inclusive of all aspects of Addiction. If this is not done, switching to use of another substance or engagement in other addictive behaviours happens commonly, with devastating consequences to individuals and families.

The American Society of Addiction Medicine (ASAM), which has become the largest professional association in North America for doctors who are interested in prevention, treatment, medical education, research, and public policy advocacy regarding Addiction and related health conditions, approved the definition of Addiction[9] in 2012 (the long definition is detailed in Appendix A). The definition was based on extensive review of current scientific work, lessons learned by experienced clinicians, and the work of experts in research and clinical practice.

DEFINITION OF ADDICTION

The short version of the definition of Addiction as outlined by ASAM, as also discussed in Chapter 1, is as follows:

> Addiction is a primary, chronic disease of brain reward, motivation, memory and related circuitry. Dysfunction in these circuits leads to characteristic biological, psychological, social and spiritual manifestations. This is reflected in an individual pathologically pursuing reward and/or relief by substance use and other behaviours.

> Addiction is characterized by inability to consistently abstain, impairment in behavioural control, cravings, diminished recognition of significant problems with one's behaviours and interpersonal

relationships, and a dysfunctional emotional response. Like other chronic diseases, Addiction often involves cycles of relapse and remission. Without treatment or engagement in recovery activities, Addiction is progressive and can result in disability or premature death.

In adopting this definition, ASAM took the historically unprecedented step for a national medical organization determining that Addiction involves the pursuit of rewards and sources of relief, and that psychoactive substances and behaviours can serve as sources of both. A key point is that ASAM's definition did not state that Addiction to various substances (alcohol, stimulants such as cocaine, hallucinogens such as marijuana) does or does not exist, or that Addiction to various behaviours (eating, spending, sexual behaviours) does or does not exist. It says that Addiction exists. It is not about drugs or addictive behaviours necessarily. It is about the brain. Specifically, it is about dysfunctions in reward and other circuitry in the brain and it defines and describes Addiction, not addictions. This definition is now endorsed by the Canadian Society of Addiction Medicine (C*SAM) and the International Society of Addiction Medicine (ISAM). The entire definition of Addiction as outlined by ASAM can be read in Appendix A.

This definition of Addiction is ground breaking in that it is the first time health care professionals have come together with a common understanding that Addiction is about more than just the substance and has many other implications for the person than just behaviour.

CHARACTERISTICS OF ADDICTION

The following explanations and case histories illustrate what has been established now from all the historical research and personal experiences to help people appreciate the depth and breadth of the disease of Addiction in its various manifestations. All the case histories use certain substances or behaviours that illustrate Addiction but these examples can be representative of all substances and addictive behaviours. The ABCDE mnemonic that follows illustrates issues related to Abstinence, Behavioural control, Craving, Diminished recognition of problems, and Emotional responses that are dysfunctional.

Abstinence. The 'inability to consistently abstain' emphasizes that short periods of abstinence are achievable for a person with Addiction. However, these periods deceptively provide reassurance to the affected individual because control does not appear to be lost. Since the disease involves impairment in the ability to recognize significant problems in life, it is hoped that this characteristic will be recognized sooner by loved ones, primary care physicians, or other professional caregivers than it may be by the person with Addiction. This way treatment can be provided earlier rather than later on when consequences begin to compound.

During periods of abstinence, some features of the disease may become inactive in day-to-day experience, including things like cravings and impairment in behavioural control. Yet the last two characteristics—the diminished recognition of life problems (which persons other than the affected individual with Addiction have no trouble recognizing) and the dysfunctional emotional response— often persist. These last two characteristics require both significant and subtle attention in recovery. This can be done using individual and group psychotherapy found in professional treatment, mutual support, and other efforts at self-help, the development of new social networks and leisure activities, and through spiritual growth. Clinically, these two areas of diminished recognition of problems and the emotional response require constant vigilance, monitoring, and accountability. It is necessary to address these issues in treatment or else recovery stability will be compromised. The continued pursuit of abstinence from all mood-altering substances and unhealthy behaviours is critical for health. Abstinence is defined by ASAM as follows:

Intentional and consistent restraint from the pathological pursuit of reward and/or relief that involves the use of substances and other behaviors. These behaviors may involve, but are not necessarily limited to, gambling, video gaming, spending, compulsive eating, compulsive exercise, or compulsive sexual behaviors.

The implications of this definition are demonstrated by Anna's case example. That is, that abstinence does not necessarily guarantee health. Likewise, struggles with abstinence do not necessarily indicate a lack of health.

Case History: Anna. *I realized very young that I had a problem with alcohol. I tried many ways to control my drinking. I changed the type of alcohol I drank. I changed when I drank. I changed how I drank, where I drank. I would quit for a while. The amount of time I was able to abstain decreased with each attempt. I started drinking every day, and earlier in the day. I was unable to abstain for longer than about twelve hours at the end of my drinking career. There were times when I would not drink for a few weeks, even months, early on. However, even then there were times when I would attempt to abstain and it would only last a few days when I had planned on not drinking for weeks. Sometimes it seemed random how long the periods of abstinence were. Looking back, even when I was abstinent from alcohol, my thinking was squirrelly. I always had underlying issues with food and relationships. I foolishly thought that if I could abstain from drinking for a few weeks, that I was still in control and everything was okay.*

Since I have stopped drinking alcohol and entered recovery, I have realized that my Addiction still manifests in my relationships with food and people. Abstinence is difficult in these areas because you have to eat and interact. I have had to set boundaries around the foods I can and cannot eat, patterns of eating, and environments that I expose myself to, like coffee shops and bakeries. Like with drinking, I have had difficulties abstaining consistently. I have had periods of healthy abstinence but also times of bingeing and purging with food. There are times when I seem to be doing well and out of the blue I end up at a coffee shop ordering three donuts that I eat in the car on the way home. This is what would happen when I was drinking. During a period of abstinence I would be feeling fine and yet find myself in the liquor store. At that moment, nothing would have stopped me from going. The mere thought that I would be going to have a drink would reduce my anxiety and I would feel high without taking a drink. I have had to set boundaries around how much I inter-act with certain individuals and look honestly at who is healthy for me. Again, I have had difficulty keeping these boundaries consistently. When I look back at my slips and relapses with food and relationships, I can sometime see warning signs, but not always. It is almost like the disease just takes over.

Although I have now managed just over three years of consistent abstinence from alcohol, I have not had consistent abstinence from the food and relationship part of my Addiction. I have come to accept that food and relationship issues will come and go in my life and the degree to which they are present is a reflection on how active my disease is. I believe my disease will always be present and that it is a part of me, but not all of me. I will not be cured. Acceptance of this actually gives me some solace and serenity.

I am very aware of how my disease manifests in my daily life. I put my recovery program first. I attend AA meetings at least twice a week and attend a group therapy session once a week. I do not put myself in environments where there is alcohol and if I end up around it, I always have a list of phone numbers or exit strategies in the back of my mind in order to protect my recovery. I do not try to be strong and prove I can be around alcohol. My disease tells me that it would be okay to be around it but I have learned that it is not healthy for me. I try to be as honest as I can about when I deviate from my food and relationship boundaries. With food, I have a system that is always evolving. There are certain foods and habits that for me are never acceptable, and others that come and go based on my level of spiritual fitness. I have to always be mindful of *whether I am being triggered to eat or whether I am actually hungry. I check with others frequently for feedback about what they are seeing.*

To manage my disease, I focus on the physical, mental, emotional, and particularly spiritual part of my program. I find regular exercise beneficial. I find it meditative and feel healthier when doing it. I find now that I am in recovery, I look at life differently. I seem to look for positives in any situation and not to 'figure out' everything and everybody. I accept people, places, and things as best I can and remind myself I have no control over them. Acceptance, for me, is the key to my sobriety. Whether through brain washing, habit, or some other means, I seem to default to looking for the positive in any situation and focus on gratitude when experiencing difficult feelings. I have learned that feelings will not kill me, and ignoring them keeps me sick. I need to feel my feelings, not judge them, and move forward as best I can. I no longer try to think my way out of everything. I have learned that I have an addictive brain and that I sometimes try to fix problems with the part of me that is damaged or broken (my brain). I find meditation very helpful, as I feel more connected with myself and the universe, and that gives me a peace and serenity that is always present to some degree. I feel it offsets the natural progression of my disease.

For Anna, the pursuit of abstinence in her recovery is apparent and she is clear about the struggles present with not only achieving abstinence, but in first defining what that looks like for her. It is possible to remove mood-altering substances like alcohol and drugs from life without any consequence. This is not possible for other aspects of life like work, exercise, sex and, in Anna's story, food and people. Just because these are part of life for every human being does not mean that they cannot become dysfunctional under the umbrella of Addiction. Therefore, being clear on motivation, or what is driving the behaviour, as well as feelings, can help give clarity on what is healthy for you. Without abstinence from all mood-altering substances, including caffeine and nicotine, the brain is still compromised and the addiction-related circuits remain active, making it harder to maintain sobriety or benefit from recovery.

Impairment in Behaviour Control. Behavioural manifestations and complications of Addiction, primarily due to impaired control can include:

a. Excessive use or engagement in addictive behaviours, at higher frequencies or quantities than intended, often associated with a persistent desire for and unsuccessful attempts at behavioural control;

b. Excessive time lost in substance use or recovering from the effects of substance use or engagement in addictive behaviours, with significant adverse impact on social and occupational functioning (e.g. the development of interpersonal relationship problems or the neglect of responsibilities at home, school, or work);

c. Continued use or engagement in addictive behaviours, despite the presence of persistent or recurrent physical or psychological problems, which may have been caused or exacerbated by substance use or related addictive behaviours;

d. A narrowing of the behavioural repertoire focusing on rewards that are part of Addiction; and

e. An apparent lack of ability or readiness to take consistent, ameliorative action despite recognition of problems.

Many believe that the difference between those who have Addiction and those who do not is the amount or frequency of alcohol and drug use and level of engagement in addictive behaviours, such as gambling or spending. In reality, a characteristic aspect of Addiction is the qualitative way in which the individual responds to exposures, stressors, and environmental cues. A pathological aspect of the way that people with Addiction pursue substance use or external rewards is that preoccupation, obsession, and pursuit of rewards persist despite the accumulation of adverse consequences.

These manifestations can occur compulsively or impulsively as a reflection of impaired control, and connect with craving.

Case History: Bob. *When I was drinking, I could not control my behaviours, even though I knew that they were inappropriate and not a true reflection of me. My emotional responses were all over the place and the behaviours that would follow were not normal for me either. When I was angry with people, particularly my wife and children, I would do things like yell, scream, and verbally abuse them, knowing at the time that it was wrong. I did not really want to do and say the things that were coming from my mouth. I would lie and manipulate anyone who got in the way of my drinking. I felt like this behaviour was immoral but I could not stop myself. I would hide bottles around the house so that I would always have a stash, just in case. When I had feelings I did not like, which were most of them, I didn't have the tools to deal with them, so I would drink. I would escape. I didn't know what else to do, so the cycle continued.*

Even today, in recovery, my behaviours are somewhat impaired some of the time because I am not fixed and my brain is not always sober, even if my body is. Certainly when I have been using, my brain runs amuck. When I'm high from food or relationships or I'm in withdrawal, I still have issues with my behaviour. I might say things to people that I normally would not, like swearing or name-calling. When engaging with certain people, feelings come up that I do not want to accept and then I fall into people pleasing. I still get trapped by thinking that if they are happy, I will be happy too. It never works but my funny brain keeps convincing me to try.

When I was still drinking, I was in a constant state of using or withdrawal. The behaviour was in control of me, not the other way around, as I would have liked to think. Since being in recovery, I still go through withdrawal from food or relationships but I would say that my behaviour is more consistent and I act more like me, or at least who I think I am today.

The biggest tool in my recovery toolkit for dealing with issues around behavioural control is acceptance. This means surrendering to and accepting my feelings, as well as people, places, and things. When I am in a place of acceptance, my behaviours tend to come from a place consistent with my being. They come from a place of honesty within myself and are in line with my values and beliefs. I have also learned that before engaging in behaviours I am unsure of, like relationships, I call someone first to discuss things and check it out. I know now that I cannot trust the information my brain is giving to me and it can be a bloody liar sometimes. With food, I tell myself that abstinence is just for today when I feel overwhelmed with the idea that I can no longer binge as a way of dealing with any pain inside of me.

When I was drinking, I engaged in behaviours that I was not really in control of, like driving drunk, falling down stairs, bumping into people, yelling, drunk phone calls and texts, and sexual relationships that were inappropriate. These would not have happened if I was sober. That being said, I still had impairment of control when not drunk because of my inability to deal with my feelings and the fact that Addiction is always present in some form or to some degree.

As Bob's story illustrates, the behaviours that are driven by the addictive mind are not representative of the person themselves. Addiction, and the feature of impairment in behavioural control, means compromising one's values and beliefs. This is a part of the disease that friends, family members, and colleagues have a difficult time appreciating, as often they believe that the hurtful words, lying, and acting out are intentional and meant to cause pain. The person with Addiction is impaired and not in control of their actions when the disease is active. This does not mean they cannot be held accountable by consequences and through boundaries, but they need not be blamed or shamed for what has happened. They are often even more upset than their family members or friends and to magnify that only pushes the shame deeper into darkness, where it festers and grows. Responsibility and accountability must be around recovery action. Expecting a person with Addiction to control their behaviour is illogical, as the 'B' characteristic of the disease illustrates. Since the disease is always present, there will be periodic struggles with maintaining consistent abstinence and impaired behavioural control, which is why accountability over recovery action is needed, not blaming, shaming, or expectations around behavioural control of the disease. In 12-step programs, step 1 specifically refers to powerlessness over addiction or specific substance and behaviour, and life becoming unmanageable as a consequence.[10]

Craving. The subjective experience of craving is impactful to people who have Addiction, who often view it as a major driving force in relapse. Individuals may experience craving as emotional, cognitive, or physiological, and the behavioural outflows of craving can be experienced as obsession, compulsion, or impulsive behaviour, which may occur seemingly inexplicably to the person. If the craving is satisfied in some other form than the original problem substance or behaviour, the person may even insist that they do not have craving or impairment in behavioural control.

Craving[11] is a word used by people with Addiction and professionals to describe the need to fulfill an obsessive desire. Craving is a part of the human condition and our brains are hardwired to appreciate and pursue pleasurable and natural rewards such as food and sex because of their survival value. When someone craves something and the desire is fulfilled, dopamine levels in the brain increase. Dopamine is a neurotransmitter that helps control the brain's reward and pleasure centres. It sends signals to the brain that tell us something feels good, which makes us want to do it again. With Addiction, the brain is wired to tolerate more dopamine and there is no shut off valve to say enough, so the individual wants more. When the reward circuits are activated, cravings for alcohol, drugs, or addictive behaviours become increasingly intense, seeking a way to get more dopamine, which may be inherently low or depleted due to excessive demand on the circuits.

Dealing with cravings is the responsibility of the brain's inhibitory circuit, which in the healthy brain leads to *stop*, *no more*, or *enough*. With Addiction, this inhibitory circuit is dysfunctional, so the addictive brain leads an individual to the opposite, which is *go* or *more*, and the cravings or desire continue to intensify until the person with Addiction gets relief, however brief.

The power of external cues to trigger cravings typically begins outside our conscious awareness. Brain imaging research has shown that cues as brief as thirty-three milliseconds can trigger the reward circuitry, which can lead to substance use or acting out. Helping an individual appreciate the cues or triggers that lead them to relapse can be challenging, as it is typically not in their conscious awareness. Cravings can be viewed as intense memories and brain imaging studies have also shown some intense brain activation when pictures that are linked to drug use (like a pipe or a white powdery substance resembling cocaine) are shown to people who have Addiction. These memories are the brain re-experiencing an event, so reliving a drug, sex, or other past-compulsive experience, can cause a serious emotional reaction. When compulsive thought revolves around a desire, craving and ritualized behaviour often evolves and the drive to appease craving connects with powerlessness over acting out and more unmanageability in one's life. With cravings, cortical areas associated with the sights, sounds, smells, and thoughts related to the event are activated in a manner similar to the initial experience.

Case History: Dana. When I was using drugs, craving was an issue all the time. Once I had a drug, it set off a craving for more that was never satisfied. It took more drugs as time went on to get high or escape. Once the drugs were wearing off in my mind and body, I seemed to crave more. If I didn't use for a few days, the craving became very intense, usually resulting in my obtaining drugs or alcohol. I can recall when I had a spell of controlled drinking, which for me meant only drinking on Fridays. By the time Friday would come, the craving would be so intense that the thought of ingesting a substance would bring relief prior to actually taking the drink or picking up a drug. I felt desperate and anxious when the cravings would come. Nothing could stop me from attempting to satisfy them. When I came to accept that I was powerless over alcohol and drugs, I chose abstinence. Once I consistently abstained and had some length of sobriety, the cravings stopped. Early in recovery, I still had cravings, but the intensity decreased as time went on. I had faith that they would stop, and I attended many AA and NA meetings and talked with other addicts in recovery, as well as counselors. I played the tape through when my brain entertained the idea of drinking and that seemed to decrease the cravings as well. Also, I stayed away from liquor stores and people or situations that seem to trigger any kind of craving. I still stay away from liquor stores and actually look away from them when I see them. I used to notice liquor stores everywhere. When my food is more active, I notice more donut shops. When I had an issue with caffeine, I noticed coffee shops. Now I stay away from things that may trigger my disease and bring up cravings, especially neighbourhoods where I used to go to score drugs.

When looking back at my early sobriety, craving must have still been present because I was soothing myself with food in a huge way. When I look back, it was like I was trying to fill myself up with something and when the drugs or alcohol were no longer an option, food took over. I understand it was partly because of the sugar content in sweets, but I feel it was bigger than that. I feel I was craving something all of my life. Now I identify that with finding a connection with myself and the universe, and my cravings seem to have decreased overall.

With food, I still have cravings and they can be intense at times. I can sometimes, in retrospect, recognize triggers, but not all the time. To reduce my chances of cravings I stay away from things like buffets and certain social situations. The degree to which I am experiencing cravings of any kind is an indication as to how active my disease is. I do believe that the craving is not just for a substance; it is more than that. At those moments, I am looking for a way to escape or ignore what is going on within myself. The answer to that, for myself, is accepting wherever I am in that instance. I recognize that what I have going on in my life right now is the best place that I can be and I will work as hard as needed to maintain that.

Cravings are a powerful part of Addiction and are the most powerful when the disease is active. With the A, B, and C features of Addiction, these drastically slow down or, as Dana found, fade almost completely in the context of abstinence and recovery. Cravings can be triggered by any of the five senses and can happen so fast, within milliseconds, that they are not even visible or observable at a conscious level. It can be difficult for people to connect with the idea of craving within themselves and many will deny having them. However, it is important to keep in mind that cravings come in many different ways and do not necessarily mean that you are fantasizing about using a substance but can also be craving escape, release, or fulfillment of fantasy.

As cravings happen so fast, it is important to minimize exposure to substances, as well as environments and people that increase vulnerability. The worst thing someone in recovery can do is test themselves by putting themselves into dangerous situations to prove the strength of their recovery. As we have been discussing, the brain never loses its vulnerability for this disease and can be activated quickly, even if the intention is to be in recovery. Cravings can be physical but they can also be psychological and come into people's dreams, with 'using dreams' being a very common experience for people in recovery, even long-term. Rather than panic about these experiences, it is important to view them as valuable information. Your brain is trying to tell you something about your vulnerability that needs to be addressed. There is a lot of opportunity in these experiences and they provide helpful reminders to be consistently diligent to one's health and recovery.

**Diminished recognition of significant problems with one's behaviours and interpersonal relationships.** In Addiction there is significant impairment in executive functioning, which manifests in problems with perception, learning, impulse control, compulsivity, and judgment. People with Addiction often have a lower readiness to change their dysfunctional behaviours despite mounting concerns expressed by significant others. They display an apparent lack of appreciation of the magnitude of cumulative problems and complications. The still developing frontal lobes of adolescents may both compound these deficits in executive functioning and predispose youngsters to engage in high-risk behaviours, including engaging in alcohol, nicotine, or other drug use. The profound drive to use substances or engage in apparently rewarding behaviours, which is seen in many people with Addiction, underscores the compulsive and avolitional aspect of this disease. In other words, there is a lack of drive to engage in healthy behaviours but an obsession and compulsion with unhealthy, rewarding ones. This is what "powerlessness" over Addiction and "unmanageability" of life refers to, as is described in step 1 of 12-step programs.

The example below describes the problems in relationships and with behaviours that can happen in the context of Addiction.

Case History: Larry. When I was acting out with pornography, masturbating, and having sex with multiple partners, I did not realize how dysfunctional most of my relationships had become. Some of the problems I minimized and some things I ignored or flat out denied. My personal relationships, particularly with family members, had become strained, distant, and dishonest. After abstaining from sexual acting out for some time, I was able to look back at certain relationships with a much clearer view. When I did realize there were problems in my relationships, I rarely thought it had anything to do with my watching porn or masturbating, as that is part of a being a young, healthy male, or so I believed. It was hard for me to see my role in the relationship problems that developed. I blamed problems on other people or situations and took little, if any, responsibility for my part.

Many people in my life, while I was having 'fun,' had distanced themselves from me and I did not realize it. Many of my relationships had changed and I was unaware until I had some sobriety. Even though friends no longer trusted me and did not share anything of any significance with me, I was unaware that it had anything to do with my behaviours. Again, even when becoming more responsible sexually, when my disease was very active I was not connected with what was going on in my relation-ships. Today, I realize that when there are problems in my relationships, I always have a part in it.

Many blind spots exist in the disease of Addiction and character-istic 'D' highlights that they exist with behaviour as well as rela-tionships. This is the fundamental reason why external support is a necessary part of the recovery process, as there will always be problems in behaviour or relationships that are not visible to the person with Addiction. As Larry described, it is hard for the person with Addiction to see clearly what is happening in their relation-ships and life, as things are being filtered through the disease and become skewed.

While the A, B, and C characteristics tend to diminish significantly in the context of abstinence and recovery (which equal sobriety), the D and E characteristics are the life-long aspects of Addiction. As Larry shared, even when abstinent, things would be happening in his relationships that he was not aware of, including distance and disconnection. Checking in with the people in your life for their per-spective on how the relationship is going is an important part of not getting trapped in 'D'. As well, it is important to process the specif-ics of situations with people in recovery or those who understand it so that they can provide feedback and highlight any disease activity they can see that the person with Addiction cannot. While situations may seem insignificant to the person who is sharing, Addiction can be seen most clearly in the details. If there is something the person with Addiction does not want to discuss or becomes reactive to, then this is an area that requires further exploration. Continuing to avoid it will only serve to reinforce disease activity. This is also very true of feelings which, in conjunction with relationships, are the most dif-ficult area for people with Addiction to explore.

Dysfunctional Emotional response. Emotional changes in Addiction can include:

a. Increased anxiety, dysphoria (feeling unwell or unhappy), and emotional pain;

b. Increased sensitivity to stressors associated with the recruitment of brain stress systems, such that 'things seem more stressful' as a result; and

c. Difficulty in identifying feelings, distinguishing between feelings and the bodily sensations of emotional arousal, and describing feelings to other people (sometimes referred to as alexithymia).

The emotional aspects of Addiction are quite complex. Some people use alcohol, drugs, or pathologically pursue other rewards because they are seeking positive reinforcement or the creation of a positive emotional state (i.e., euphoria). Others pursue substance use or other rewards because they experience relief from negative emotional states (i.e. dysphoria), which is negative reinforcement.

Beyond the initial experiences of reward and relief, there is a dysfunctional emotional state present in most cases of Addiction that is associated with the persistence of engagement with addictive behaviours. The state of Addiction is not the same as the state of intoxication. When anyone experiences mild intoxication through the use of alcohol or other drugs, or when one engages non-pathologically in potentially addictive behaviours such as gambling or eating, one may experience a high. This is felt as a positive emotional state associated with increased dopamine and opioid peptide activity in reward circuits in the brain.

After such an experience, there is a neurochemical rebound, in which the reward function does not simply revert to baseline, but often drops below the original levels as the brain tries to re-establish homeostasis. This is usually not consciously perceptible by the individual and is not necessarily associated with functional impairments. Over time, however, repeated experiences with substance use or addictive behaviours are not associated with ever-increasing reward circuit activity and are not as subjectively rewarding. Our brains reach a limit in terms of how much pleasure something can give, which creates a lot of frustration for the person who is trying to catch the intensity of that first high.

When a person experiences withdrawal from drug use or comparable behaviours, there is an anxious, agitated, dysphoric, and labile emotional experience, related to suboptimal reward and the recruitment of brain and hormonal stress systems. The brain is not happy that it is no longer being hit with these feel good chemicals, whether they were externally introduced by ingesting substance or internally initiated through behaviour engagement like sex or gambling. While tolerance develops to the high, it does not develop to the emotional low associated with the cycle of intoxication and withdrawal. This low never becomes easier or acceptable.

Thus, in Addiction, people repeatedly attempt to create a high, but what they mostly experience is a deeper low. Those with Addiction feel a compulsive need to use substance or behaviour to try to resolve their dysphoric emotional state and their physiological symptoms of withdrawal. People with Addiction get to the point of using to function and feel normal, as well as to avoid these lows, rather than to feel good. The resetting of homeostasis or balance through physiological or behaviour change is called allostasis. Although people from any background, with or without Addiction, may choose to get high, it is important to appreciate that Addiction is not solely a function of choice but driven by this complicated process of reward and relief happening in the brain. Simply put, Addiction is not a desired condition.

Emotions arise at the place where mind and body meet; they are the body's reaction to the mind. If there is a conflict between thought and emotion, the thought will be the lie and the emotion will be the relative truth about how you feel at that time. It is essential not to judge feelings or thoughts because of this; rather, we need to pay attention to them as they carry valuable information about the self. The example below illustrates how the emotional relationship can become very dysfunctional in active disease.

Case History: Amanda. *When I was binging or purging with food, my emotional responses were dysfunctional. I would overreact to situations as well as under-react. I would become angry or sad for no real reason. There were times when my children would be fighting and I did not react at all, as if I did not care. Intellectually, I would know what to do to discipline them, but emotionally I could not react. During periods of withdrawal, my emotional response was dysfunctional as well. I remember family and friends sharing their concern about my eating with me, I could hear the words but my mind would not allow me to react. Almost like there was a cement wall around that emotional part of myself that did not want me to feel, probably because then I would see the truth and want to change.*

I'm not sure what exactly happened to make the shift from disease to recovery, but slowly I began to see that what I was doing was not working for me anymore. I did not want to feel like a robot just going through the motions, I wanted to live and experience things. I wanted to not just feel good but to feel something. The awareness of my feelings was hard and even a few years into my recovery some of them are still really hard to look at, particularly my shame and anger. I can get easily hooked back into these feelings without even realizing it, but the difference is now I can pull back from them usually by talking it out or writing about it.

When I think back to before I was in recovery, my emotional responses to situations were not always congruent with what I was thinking, or my beliefs and values. I was not acting as I felt inside. My inability to deal with my feelings in the past led to inappropriate emotional responses as well as problems with behavioural control. I believe this is all linked together. Working my recovery program as established with my treatment team of peers, therapist, and physician helps me accept my feelings, which results in more appropriate emotional responses as well as appropriate and congruent behaviour despite the initial dysfunctional response that may be triggered.

In addition to worries about substance use or problem behaviours, the challenges with feelings that come with Addiction is the second most cited concern for people surrounding the sufferer, and sometimes of the person themselves. These challenges can include anger outbursts, suicidal ideation, overreaction, under-reaction, being numb and cold, and emotional unpredictability. Many people believe that these feelings-based challenges are the direct result of the substance use or problematic behaviours, such that if the person would just stop using, they would become emotionally healthy. This is not the case. Emotional health in the context of Addiction is a major component of the recovery work that is needed and takes time and effort to explore and develop. Identification of, connection with, and healthy expression of feelings does not come easily or naturally to people with Addiction and takes time, patience and understanding from everybody. Feelings are a major driver of this disease and need to be regarded with the importance they carry, without falling into the trap that emotional dysfunction is all down to the brain being high or intoxicated. In reality, emotional dysfunction is the second life-long, persistent part of the disease and, as such, needs to be discussed and explored, not feared. Feelings do not kill us; they provide valuable information, but will kill the person with Addiction if they continue to be numbed and avoided.

The implications of the ABCDE characteristics are profound. It is now recognized that the problems in brain function likely lead to individuals persistently engaging in addictive behaviours and using substances pathologically in the first place, and further complications arise over time that make Addiction treatment and recovery difficult. Hence, substances are an aggravating factor for the disease of Addiction long term. They are not the causative factor, especially when one appreciates that abstinence from the substance is a starting step for recovery, not the end step. Further, we have come to appreciate that recovery can begin even prior to abstinence being established with harm reduction measures as a means to engage individuals and help them towards their healing journey towards health.

CHAPTER SUMMARY

Historically, the word Addiction has not been widely used as a medical diagnosis and, to date, there continues to be stigma attached to the words 'addict' and 'addiction,' which is why we have set out to change the language to 'person with Addiction' or 'person in recovery' and 'Addiction.' In 2011, ASAM, the largest professional association in North America for doctors who are interested in prevention, treatment, medical education, research, and advocacy of public policy regarding Addiction and related health conditions, approved a definition of Addiction (Appendix A). It was based on extensive review of current scientific work, lessons learned by experienced clinicians, and experts in research and clinical practice. This definition is now endorsed by C*SAM (Canadian Society of Addiction Medicine) and the International Society of Addiction Medicine (ISAM).

The definition of Addiction recognizes the primary and chronic nature of the brain disease that involves reward, motivation, memory, and related circuitry. The characteristic biological, psychological, social, and spiritual manifestations need to be explored by individuals affected so that the pathological pursuing of reward and/or relief by substance use and other behaviours can be addressed.

The characteristics of Addiction as illustrated by inability to consistently **a**bstain, impairment in **b**ehavioural control, **c**raving, **d**iminished recognition of significant problems with one's behaviours and interpersonal relationships, and a dysfunctional **e**motional response require a lot of attention in treatment and recovery. As Addiction often involves cycles of relapse and remission, like other chronic diseases, a continuing care framework is required in recovery. Although Addiction is progressive and can result in disability or premature death, with proper treatment, meaning abstinence in the context of holistic recovery (which equals sobriety), a high quality of life is possible, more so than with any other chronic disease.

Chapter 3: Addictive Thinking

This chapter examines the features of addictive thinking, which is how Addiction manifests at the cognitive level, as well as how addictive thinking affects recovery and precedes relapse. We also explore the value of increasing self-awareness to mitigate addictive thinking and discuss the impact of self-talk as a recovery tool.

Distortion in thought,[1] or abnormal thinking, was first recognized in Alcoholics Anonymous and labelled "stinking thinking". Distortion in thinking, also coined 'addictive thinking' by Dr. Abraham Twerski in 1997, is not unique to Addiction. Everyone can be challenged by cognitive distortions. This typically occurs when people feel insecure, have low self-esteem, feel stressed, and have difficulty adjusting to life's challenges. When life becomes too challenging, there is an increased desire to escape or become numb. Addictive thinking does not necessarily indicate Addiction, but the intensity and regularity of it is most common among people with the disease.

Addictive thinking has logic that can be very seductive and misleading, but it is not based in reality. For instance, the person with Addiction may think that today when they drink they can stop at two drinks even though the historical evidence is they drink to black out at fifteen or more drinks. Addictive thinking says that this time will be different, which of course it is not the reality. The person is not consciously misleading others, although this may occur, yet they are unable to stop because of Addiction. Typically, people with Addiction are taken in by their own thinking, actually deceiving themselves, and it takes someone from the outside to point this out and challenge the distortion. This may not always be welcomed, but only then can people with Addiction start to appreciate their addictive thinking and change their misperception of reality to be more realistic. As in the above example, realizing that one drink is too many because one is never enough.

The two key aspects of addictive thinking are: obsession and control. Obsessive thoughts crowd out all others and become the most dominant, which drains mental energy. These can intrude at any time. It is also important to be aware that obsession is not limited to substances or behaviours. People with Addiction may find themselves obsessing about turning off lights before they leave home, if their children are safe, numbers, world events, reading, or any other number of things. Attempts to control or get rid of the obsessions only increase their intensity. For an example, try this exercise: Do *not* think about a pink elephant. Whatever you do, do not think about a pink elephant. Just stop. Do not do it.

Well? What image popped into your brain? If you are like most people, the image of a pink elephant flooded in quickly, if not instantly when you were told not to think of one. Trying to control or get rid of an obsessive thought is like trying to swim against a current. Our brains have a difficult time distinguishing between 'do' and 'do not' commands, so the debate of 'do I or don't I?' becomes perceived as 'do, do, do'. Just like water flowing in a river, thoughts and feelings will go by if they are left alone. Obsession sets the stage for addictive thinking and control is the trap that keeps one stuck in it and acting out from it.

Addictive thinking has also been described as a person making unhealthy decisions without realizing the harm in the moment. For example, one can start with the thought of 'I need money' and then decide to go to the casino and play the slot machines for eight hours, convinced that it is their turn to win to satisfy their goal of obtaining money. A person with Addiction will often build a case for this story such as 'I will win this time', without any supporting evidence for the thought being rational.

Another interesting characteristic of addictive thinking is that it usually does not affect the ability to spot problems in others, only in oneself. This means that people experiencing addictive thinking are able to see others more objectively than themselves. For people with Addiction, the self-concept is clouded by self-doubt and low self-esteem which puts up a barricade to seeing the self honestly, yet they can spot things in others that they are experiencing. For example, the person with Addiction can readily spot unhealthy using or identify excuses to getting well. However, when challenged on these characteristics in themselves they deny it, because they cannot see it. To understand how Addiction operates, it is important to understand additional key aspects of addictive thinking.

FEATURES OF ADDICTIVE THINKING

Addictive thinking is the conglomeration of irrational, distorted thoughts. It perpetuates exaggerated or irrational thought patterns that prolong the effects of psychological states, especially depression and anxiety. It can generate feelings of chaos and anxiety internally, which adds to the discomfort of Addiction. Addictive thinking starts with an initial thought that quickly snowballs.

Addictive thinking is black or white, all or nothing, it does not live in the gray zone. When someone has all-or-nothing thinking, they have the tendency to do something to the extreme or not at all and they have difficulty seeing the other options that may be available to them. This type of thinking leads many people with Addiction to label themselves as 'lazy' or 'procrastinators' because they struggle to find a realistic balance for achieving goals. For example, the goal may be to become physically healthy. To the addictive thinker, the options are extreme dieting with intense exercise seven days a week, or else staying in the same routine of eating lots of junk and processed food with no exercise. If one can move beyond addictive thinking, one realizes that starting to walk three times per week and cutting out a nightly snack are realistic places to start in moving towards this goal. Addiction is a disease of more, so one has to be careful when establishing goals that they are truly balanced or else one may quickly find themselves in extreme behavioural patterns. Unfortunately the extreme options are not sustainable and lead to burn out, which can increase feelings of shame and low self-worth.

With all-or-nothing addictive thinking, it becomes easy to focus on what is not happening or working well and to become disconnected from recovery action. The mind may think 'I must do it perfectly or not at all' or 'I feel so much better now that I've been abstinent for three months, I don't need to do anymore 12-step meetings.' In relationships, all-or-nothing thinking can perpetuate negativity and self-doubt in thoughts such as, 'My partner was so insensitive today and they obviously do not love me.' These thoughts are not true, but they are accepted as truth internally. The more a person thinks in extremes, the more difficulty they will have coping with everyday reality. In healthy or non-addictive thinking, one can see all the available options and think in shades of gray, not just extremes.

Rationalization, denial, projection, and minimization are all psychological strategies that take place in the unconscious mind to distort reality and maintain a socially acceptable self-image. Healthy people use similar defenses throughout life as coping mechanisms to reduce anxiety but with active Addiction these defense mechanisms become significantly heightened. Progressive elimination of them is critical for a person with Addiction to stay in healthy recovery and decrease their vulnerability to relapse.

Rationalization occurs when a person's true motivation is concealed and they reason with themselves and others that something makes sense and is a good idea. An example of rationalization is thinking that having one drink of alcohol after being in recovery for ten years is safe. 'It is safe because I have not had any cravings for alcohol in years, am not bothered being around it, and have done a lot of work on myself in recovery.' Unfortunately these ideas are created by the addictive mind and used to seek reward or relief which, ultimately, feeds the disease, not recovery.

The defense mechanism of projection is placing the blame on others rather than oneself, such that the person is not being accountable for their actions. In active Addiction, this could sound like, 'You would use too if you had a spouse like mine.' Projection can also involve placing feelings onto other people that you are experiencing yourself, for instance, identifying a friend as being angry, even though they are not, when it is really you that is angry.

Denial is an automatic and unconscious response people have when feeling threatened, whether this is real or perceived. Rationalization and projection reinforce denial as an individual justifies, in a seemingly logical manner, unhealthy behaviours to avoid the truth. For example, the use of pornography and masturbation may be justified by someone because they feel that it is because their spouse is not as sexually available as they would like. In reality, engagement in pornography and masturbation are likely to make them *less* interested in sex with their spouse and/or create tension between them, making a sexual relationship unsatisfactory. In denial, a person minimizes the harm being done to themselves or others, as it is too difficult to face this reality. This is why active Addiction occurs for much longer than family members expect it will. Denial sparks a lot of anger from others: 'Can't they see what this is doing to him/her/us?' The struggling person with Addiction may want to change and sees consequences to their actions, but are overwhelmed by and entrenched in their disease. With denial, the part of the brain suffering from Addiction sends strong messages that everything is okay. The defense mechanism of minimization often goes hand-in-hand with denial. It lessens the perceived consequences of Addiction, including the impact on self and others. It is a form of avoidance that feeds into denial. Minimization can sound like 'things aren't so bad,' 'what's the big deal?' or 'I'm fine.'

When achieving pleasure or relieving discomfort becomes a major goal of life, people often turn to substances or behaviours that provide this instant gratification or relief. Our culture embraces addictive thinking and encourages instant gratification. Addictive thinking precedes the behavioural part of Addiction and precipitates all relapse behaviours, as illustrated further by this case example.

Case History: Francis. *Francis, a thirty-three-year-old woman, sought help after her last relapse. In describing the relapse, she explained how she was invited on a date with a guy whom she had liked for several weeks. They had met at work but since they were in different departments, knew very little about each other. On the date they went to a fancy restaurant and he asked Francis if she wanted red or white wine with dinner. She wanted to tell him she didn't drink and knew she should, but told herself that there would be no harm in having a glass or two of wine with dinner, as her problem drinking was when she was alone at home. Francis only had two glasses with dinner and was able to control her drinking during the date, but she was in denial and minimized the risk. She continued to drink when she got home that evening and this continued for the next three days. Thankfully Francis was able to see the risks inherent in this relationship and decided to take a hiatus from dating to continue working on her recovery and self. As she prepared to start dating again, she realized the importance of disclosing to partners before going out that she does not drink and is in recovery as she has no desire to start off a relationship with dishonesty.*

Francis' story provides an illustration of what rationalization can sound like and the devastating impact it can have. Denial cannot only perpetuate relapse, it also makes it more difficult for the person to re-enter recovery, as their minimization, rationalization, and denial work together to keep them entrenched in seeking immediate relief, reward, or escape rather than seeing the damage the behaviours are causing to them and those around.

Morbid expectations, also known as catastrophizing, are when an individual is anticipating that the worst will happen. Sometimes this occurs as an emotional coping strategy; if one expects the worst then they will not be disappointed. Morbid expectations can lead to hypervigilance, as one is always planning for the worst possible outcomes and thinking up ways to control or prevent the situation. People with Addiction are obviously not the only ones who worry and anticipate the worst, but they tend to do this more frequently than others since it is a feature of addictive thinking. Even when things are going well, people with Addiction have a tendency to feel burdened by morbid expectations and may sabotage the situation because they feel undeserving of things going well. For example, picking a fight with a romantic partner because they believe the relationship is going to end anyway. Many people with Addiction will describe themselves as 'self-sabotaging', which is not an accurate description. Rather, their Addiction is what encourages them to seek a destructive outcome in life, as this way the Addiction is more likely to be reinforced through escape. Thus, it is not the person that is purposefully out to sabotage a situation, but rather it is a consequence of their disease. The self-sabotage is a symptom of Addiction rather than a personality flaw.

Addiction is a brain disease affecting memory circuitry, which alters the perception of time. Periods of abstinence lasting for hours, days, or weeks may prove to the person with Addiction that abstinence is possible any time. One of the most common phrases heard in active disease is 'I can quit anytime.' This is not the case, as people with Addiction are unable to stop any time they wish—otherwise, they likely would have already. Family and friends can see this but, unfortunately, the person in active Addiction cannot. This can cause a lot of conflict with loved ones. It is important to appreciate that time is variable for everyone and, at times, minutes may feel endless, while at other times, hours and days can fly by. The person with Addiction's version of time may be skewed compared to others and he or she may believe there has been a lengthy period of abstinence when it has really been two days. In recovery, the emphasis is to take it one day, hour, or minute at a time, as it can become overwhelming to look beyond this, especially in the first three to six months of sobriety. 'Time takes time' is a phrase used in treatment to convey the importance of patience and staying in the process with recovery. It is not an immediate endpoint or finite destination, but an ongoing path of discovery. This is particularly challenging for a person with Addiction who has intolerance of delay and carries the need for instant gratification. We all live in a culture that fuels the addictive concept of time, the need for instant gratification, and intolerance for delay. With technology, people can instantly find what they need and connect with others in seconds. There may be some irritation or frustrations when needs are not met quickly.

Hypersensitivity is another feature of addictive thinking and results in the person being reactive and emotional in situations where these reactions seem unwarranted or exaggerated. We have all witnessed someone who has become angry in a benign situation, like when they are emptying a dishwasher or driving in traffic, and wondered what their problem was. Even if we know the individual, we may not understand what is driving that reaction or understand their dysfunctional emotional response, as we would perhaps not react the same way to that situation. Some people are more sensitive or vulnerable to stress and tend to feel emotional discomfort more acutely than others. Just as some people with fair skin are more sensitive to sun exposure and burn when others tan, some people have greater emotional sensitivity when encountering conflict, stress, and discomfort. According to Dr. Twerski, a person with Addiction's emotional sensitivity may be similar to someone with a sunburn, who feels more pain with simple touch because their skin is already irritated and pain sensitive because of the sunburn. A situation that might provoke a strong reaction because of pre-existing sensitivity in some may not provoke a reaction in others because they do not have that vulnerability.

It is important to appreciate that Addiction is about the pursuit of reward or high, but it is also about relief from negative feelings in an attempt to feel normal. When someone is hypersensitive, there is often an increased desire to escape or numb the overwhelming and uncomfortable feelings. A young woman in early recovery once shared with us that it felt like all her feelings were in high definition (HD) and she was struggling to remain balanced as she preferred a low definition world. Hypersensitivity tends to lessen over time with active recovery. Emotional stability in the midst of stress and chaos is an indicator of health, self-confidence, and solid recovery.

With Addiction, people frequently feel tremendous shame, which is different from guilt. Guilt occurs when someone feels remorse for something they have done, and shame occurs when someone feels less than they are. Guilt can lead to corrective action but shame can be toxic and typically leads to resignation and despair. Shame can be generated from many things, including our culture, upbringing, and genetic makeup. Everyone has experienced shame at some point in his or her life, which can be identified as when we do not feel good enough or worthy. With Addiction, feelings of low self-esteem and shame tend to be more severe and circumstances that may invoke guilt in an emotionally healthy person invoke shame in a person with Addiction. For example, Emily was helping her friend move. She accidentally dropped and broke her friend's precious sculpture. She immediately felt guilty for not paying more attention, making a conscious effort to be more careful in the future. If she had felt shame, Emily would have beaten herself up and blamed herself for being so careless and thoughtless. It could have potentially wrecked her mood for the rest of the day, blowing the situation out of perspective. When people with Addiction understand and accept that they have a disease, shame can shift to guilt. It is easier to process guilt and come to a place of acceptance than it is with shame. While people with Addiction need to be fully responsible for their recovery, they are not at fault for having this disease. If Emily can realize she is human and makes mistakes, she can process her feelings of guilt about breaking the sculpture without taking the event on personally and seeing it as a reflection of her failure as a person.

The illusion of being in control and the belief that 'I can do it on my own' is a challenging step to overcome. When people with Addiction insist that they can control their substance use or compulsive behaviour despite evidence to the contrary, this is the delusion of control. This leads to people drinking again after years of sobriety with the rationalization of 'I can keep it at one this time', or 'It will be different now,' when in fact their lives have become unmanageable and they are powerless over their Addiction.

The feeling of being in charge, of having a say over what happens in one's life, is beneficial for the achievement of life goals. Having self-confidence, also known as mastery with self-regulation, is about discipline and personal accountability. It must not to be confused with control. Everyone falls somewhere along the continuum of control and it is a bigger issue for some, while not so much for others. For many people, control can be an issue that gets in the way, especially with the more stressful aspects of life. With Addiction, the desire for control goes awry and becomes a trap. The inability to admit impairment in control or the inability to control everything, which is often seen as manipulation by others, is characteristic of addictive thinking. With Addiction, the delusion of control must first be overcome for a person in recovery to admit and accept powerlessness over their disease. It is essential to acknowledge the power of Addiction to be able to surrender and discover personal power through recovery.

There are many reasons that lead us to control. People's beliefs and feelings lead them to control others, certain situations, money, communication, food, workflow, the environment, and other important aspects of our world. Typically, there are three underlying feelings behind someone's controlling tendencies: fear, unworthiness, and distrust. With fear, there is worry that things will not turn out as hoped or that something bad will happen. With unworthiness, people convince themselves that they do not deserve support and that things will not go their way and, instead, that they deserve to suffer. With distrust, people may be scared to let go and count on others, as it has not worked out well in the past. People begin to believe that they have to manage every aspect of the situation, relationship, or conversation; otherwise, it will not go the way they want. In reality, everyone needs to rely on faith, their self-worth and trust in others to move forward in life.

ADDICTIVE THINKING AND RECOVERY

Holistic recovery is a framework for developing awareness of addictive thinking and lessening the impact it has on daily living. A goal of treatment with addictive thinking is to increase awareness of distorted perceptions, talk about feelings, and take recovery action. Awareness alone is not enough; it is the commitment to recovery action that in turn creates more awareness and change, which are necessary for growth.

Journaling,[2] relaxation,[3] and meditation[4] are effective tools to deal with the chaos of the mind. Journaling is a way to process feelings and help gain clarity about disease thinking. Journaling is a powerful tool for helping us work through our thoughts. Thinking about something gives us many ideas, but it is often in the writing of those ideas that we can start to see patterns emerge. Through these patterns, people begin to discover who they really are and change the things in life that are not working. In addition, journaling helps people keep track of their insights, making it a continual process in which they enhance, refine, and expand ideas and helps identify the things that may be holding them back. It also helps people understand how to address these issues in a positive, concrete way. Writing about stressful events helps one come to terms with them, thus reducing the impact of these stressors on overall health. When feelings and thoughts are bottled up for too long, people can become ill due to the adverse effects on the immune system. The field of psychoneuroimmunology is devoted to the study of these connections.

To get healthy and stay that way, people generally have to get to the root of their repressed feelings and release them. Writing helps remove mental blocks and allows people to use their brainpower to better understand themselves, others, and the world.

Journaling will be most effective if done daily for approximately twenty minutes. Begin anywhere and forget about spelling and punctuation. Privacy is necessary if you are to write without censor. Write quickly, as this frees your brain from 'shoulds' and other blocks to successful journaling. If it helps, pick a theme for the day, week, or month (for example, peace of mind, confusion, change, or anger). The most important rule of all is that there are no rules. Appendix B outlines how to journal effectively.

There are many techniques for relaxation and meditation. The terms are sometimes used interchangeably but they are distinct experiences, even though meditation leads to relaxation. Relaxation methods are designed to help a person to attain a state of increased calmness and reduce levels of anxiety, stress, or anger. With relaxation, the goal is to achieve a conscious, slow relaxation of all the major muscle groups and activity of the body to stimulate the relaxation response. This includes deeper, slower breathing, decreased muscle tension, lowered blood pressure, and lowered heart rate, among other health benefits. Typically when the body starts to relax, the mind follows suit with diminished obsessive and racing thoughts.

Meditation can be accompanied by varying degrees of relaxation but that is not the goal, only a side effect. Meditation is a mental discipline by which the individual creates an intention to move beyond the thinking mind into a deeper, more profound state of awareness and transcendental state. There are numerous benefits to meditation, including but not limited to better self-knowledge, clarity of thought, lowered stress, improved physical health, greater focus, and overall wellbeing. There are other practices that people may call meditation, such as contemplation, which is reflecting on positive thoughts, and concentration, which involves focusing the mind on specific ideas. Contemplation and concentration are more focused on control or substitution of thoughts, whereas true meditation is a process of letting go, acceptance, and aligning with the functioning of the universe. Control or substitution can bring temporary relief by shifting the focus; however, true relief only comes with a discipline that involves acceptance of all that is without judgment or desire to fix. This acceptance also connects with equanimity, which allows one to not get caught in judgment with labelling things 'good' or 'bad'. With equanimity there is a true balance in the self.

ADDICTIVE THINKING AND RELAPSE

It has been consistently observed by professionals and people with Addiction that addictive thinking precedes addictive behaviours and precipitates relapse. With all relapses, the pattern starts with a spiritual disconnection and, over time, builds up. This is the relapse continuum.

Spirituality is the discovery of our authentic self without the trimmings or labels of religion, which gives us a rich source of values and deeper meaning in life. Spiritual relapse begins when there is loss of meaning and distortion in values. It usually occurs in the context of disconnection from oneself and others. There is a tendency with spiritual relapse to lose hope and faith, while being caught in fighting and trying to control the disease.

Emotional relapse then occurs. In the face of fighting powerlessness, feelings of shame, resentment, impatience, blame, hopelessness, and feeling victimized arise. People with Addiction increasingly have difficulty sitting with their feelings and default to avoidance and minimization.

Mental or cognitive relapse occurs with an increase in addictive thinking as well as negative self-talk, worry, and analysis of emotional problems rather than feeling the feelings. Most of us have become conditioned to believe that people need to always be thinking about something, but a large proportion of thoughts are repetitive, useless, and can be harmful. Thinking too much is also a rather insidious way of avoiding dealing with feelings that may not always be obvious.

If an individual is unaware of these relapse warning signs, they will continue down the slippery slope and eventually act out or use. Often people are puzzled by what precipitated their relapse but addictive thinking provides information about how active the disease is. It is often difficult to identify addictive thinking in oneself; therefore, the importance of connecting with trusted friends, family, people in healthy recovery, and health care professionals who understand Addiction is essential.

Resistance to change is also associated with addictive thinking. Health care providers need to present evidence of a person's self-defeating logic to help them establish better awareness of addictive thinking. This is essential in maintaining abstinence and promoting ongoing recovery.

INCREASING SELF-AWARENESS

As Addiction is a brain disease, some of an individual's thoughts will be driven by it too. This means that not all thinking can be trusted in the person who has Addiction. The disease of Addiction uses addictive thinking to its advantage to reinforce feelings of shame and low self-worth by amplifying destructive thinking. It sabotages thinking and feeling and revolves around the predominant belief that 'I am bad.' If you are struggling to identify what is the disease and what is you, the most prudent thing to do is talk to others and check it out with people in recovery or those you trust who understand Addiction. Talking and getting feedback is valuable to increase self-awareness, as everyone has blind spots that they may be unable to see but that others can.

The Johari Window[5] is a helpful construct used in treatment to increase self-awareness and illustrate this concept of openness and blind spots. This was created by psychologists Joseph Luft and Harrington Ingham to help people understand their relationships with themselves and others. Luft and Ingham called their construct 'Johari' by combining parts of their first names. The Johari Window (Figure 1) is illustrated as a 2x2 grid. It distinguishes what people can or cannot see in themselves and what others can or cannot see in them. It is useful to increase self-awareness, personal development, and interpersonal relationships. The Johari Window focuses on four basic aspects of the self: The public self (open); the private hidden self (secret); the blind self (blind spots); and the undiscovered self (unknown).

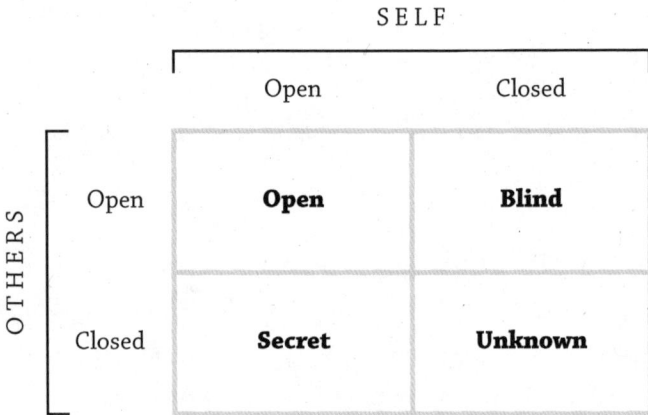

SELF

	Open	Closed
Open	**Open**	**Blind**
Closed	**Secret**	**Unknown**

OTHERS

FIGURE 1 THE JOHARI WINDOW

The *public/open self* is what you and others see. You typically do not mind discussing this part of yourself with others, as it is readily apparent already. You may not always like what is in the public/open sphere, but hopefully can work towards acceptance. A goal of individual and group therapy is to increase the size of the open area by decreasing the blind spots. This is done through being receptive to feedback. The size of the open area can also be expanded by disclosure of information, feelings, and thoughts to others. Also, people can help a person expand their open area and lessen the secret area by asking more about them. This is a goal for healthy, holistic recovery. Life and self becomes transparent, as there is no longer a need for deceit, lying, or manipulation.

The *hidden or secret self* is what you see in yourself but others do not. In this part, you hide things that are private about you as you may not want this information to be disclosed for your own protection. It could also be that you are ashamed of these areas and of having your faults and dysfunctions exposed. For example, that you have Addiction or have been unfaithful to your spouse in the past. A goal of therapy is to move hidden information, thoughts, and feelings into the open area through the process of disclosure. The aim is to disclose and expose relevant information, thoughts, and feelings with people who are safe, thereby increasing the open area. By telling others how you feel, you reduce the hidden area and increase the open area, which enables better understanding and trust. With Addiction, the disease is trying to protect itself, which is often shame-driven. People are as sick as their secrets.

The *blind self* is what is known about someone by others, but is unknown to the person. This blind area is not an effective or productive space for individuals or groups. This blind area could also be referred to as ignorance about oneself, or issues in which one is deluded. A blind area could also include issues that others are deliberately withholding from a person. By seeking or soliciting feedback from others, the aim is to reduce this area and thereby increase the open area to increase self-awareness. Others can see and hear addictive thinking and behaviour and feedback is important, whether the individual is open to it or not.

The *undiscovered or unknown self* is what you cannot see, nor can others around you. In this pane of the window, there may be good and bad things that are out of the awareness of others and yourself. Examples of unknown factors include a natural ability or aptitude that a person does not realize they possess; an unconscious fear or aversion; repressed or subconscious feelings; or conditioned behaviours or attitudes from childhood. The processes by which this information and knowledge can be uncovered are various and can be prompted through self-discovery, observation by others, or collectively through mutual discovery within a group setting. Counselling helps uncover unknown issues when therapeutically appropriate. As with disclosure and soliciting feedback, the process of self-discovery is a sensitive one. The extent and depth to which an individual is able to seek out and discover their unknown feelings are at the individual's own discretion. Some people are more keen and able than others to do this. The unknown area could also include repressed or subconscious feelings rooted in formative events and traumatic past experiences, which can stay unknown for a lifetime. With Addiction, the individual is being deceived by their brain and everyone around them is fooled too, and it can lead to lying for no reason, or not even being aware that one is lying. Things are hidden from awareness, for example, someone saying, 'I tried to call to tell you I would be late,' though no call was made.

SELF-TALK

Imagine you are working on a project while listening to the radio. When your favourite song comes on, you sing along, paying attention to the words and music. As the song ends, the broadcast turns to commercials and the DJ begins talking about the latest news and weather. You continue to work on your project and become immersed in the details of your work, oblivious to the radio that continues to emit sound. Another song comes on later and you snap to attention, returning your ears to the radio that has been playing all along.

Much like the radio, our internal thoughts and dialogue are constantly playing, sometimes in the background and sometimes in the foreground. People are not aware of all the hundreds of thoughts they have in a day, yet they still have an impact on health, feelings, and wellbeing. Self-talk is a valuable tool for health and wellness development, including as part of recovery from Addiction, and developing awareness and taking action with it can lead to benefits in many areas, including dealing with stress more effectively, exploring feelings honestly, and improving self-worth and esteem.

Self-talk[6] is the term used to refer to the ongoing, internal conversation that people have with themselves. Self-talk can focus on anything that is encountered in life, from logistical details to historical facts to relationships. Self-talk can also be instructional and used to help walk through tasks. For example, people can internally coach themselves through paying a bill online as they walk through the steps of opening up a computer, entering the password, indicating the amount of money to be paid that month, writing down the confirmation number, logging off, and shutting down the computer. Whether people are aware or not, this whole process has been guided by internal dialogue, or self-talk. Therefore, if you can learn to tune in to this dialogue and use it more effectively to reach your health and wellness goals, it can be a valuable tool that naturally exists within you.

The relationship between self-talk and other aspects of self, namely behaviour, thoughts, and feelings, is not linear. This is the reason that exploring and making changes to self-talk, particularly destructive and self-defeating patterns, can produce change in behaviour, thoughts, or feelings. An important point to keep in mind is that while you may believe your self-talk has a direct impact on the world around you, in reality it has no impact on anyone but you. You may have heard the Buddha quotation, "Holding onto anger is like drinking poison and expecting the other person to die." The same could be said of self-talk. Part of us may believe that by ruminating about a person, problem, or situation, it will create change but, in reality, it does nothing but wear our internal energy down. Since people cannot shut off their self-talk for prolonged periods as they can the radio, you need to learn ways of shifting it in directions that support health and wellness or learning to disengage from it, like in meditation, rather than maintaining thoughts that feed into chaos and disease. Avoiding or agreeing with thinking that is not accurate, like the belief that you are unworthy or a failure, has a detrimental impact on health and, in the context of Addiction, aggravates the disease and distracts from recovery. While it may bring up fear or anxiety to honestly explore this internal dialogue, ultimately this exploration will bring you closer to recovery and contentment.

You may be wondering how something like self-talk, a natural process that occurs within us, can bring one closer to serenity and improve recovery. Self-talk can support healthy levels of self-esteem and self-worth, which serve as the antidote to the powerful feeling of shame that Addiction generates in great quantities. If someone is living in shame, likely they are having thoughts generated through their self-talk that support this feeling. For example, that they cannot do anything right, are a waste of space, or that everything they touch falls apart. This is where self-talk, particularly if not honestly attended to, can erode self-worth and perpetuate low self-esteem, shame, anxiety, depression, and many other uncomfortable feelings.

As people grow up, they hear messages, both direct and indirect, from those around them. Without knowing it, they take on some of these messages as their own. This means that they hear these words or statements in their minds and cannot distinguish their internal voice from the external voice; they have merged into one. People therefore think that what they heard from others is an accurate reflection of reality and the mind supports this through self-talk. However, if people are raised in environments where there is dysfunction, disease, mental health issues, or unrealistic messages, the mind still takes on some or all of the feedback they heard as internal 'truths' that become a part of the self's definition.

When exploring self-talk, people will often be surprised to realize that a message they give to themselves is something that they heard from someone in their past. For example, every time Samantha would drop crumbs, spill a drink, or make a mess as a child, her father would say, 'Geez Samantha, get it together.' At age forty-five, every time she had a clumsy moment, she would tell herself, 'Geez Samantha, get it together.' This situation would trigger a strong feeling of shame and low self-worth within her during these moments of imperfection (i.e., being human). Over time, she began to have clarity on what messages were hers, meaning statements that she truly believed were reflective of who she is, rather than messages that were others, or based on other people's perceptions, which may not be entirely accurate. This process allows one to get closer to their personal truth and, over time, builds a foundation of self, raising esteem and worth in the process. This is a slow process that takes time and conscious effort to build, as it has taken people years to get to where they are today with their self-talk and internal dialogue. However, it is something that can be changed and have tremendous benefit, because as self-worth increases, uncomfortable feelings diminish. Healthy self-talk is a valuable tool for dealing with challenging situations as well as these uncomfortable feelings.

Addiction, being a brain disease, affects many aspects of self, including thinking. The disease of Addiction uses self-talk to its advantage by reinforcing feelings of shame and low self-worth. It does this by amplifying the 'shoulda, coulda, woulda' talk and focusing on what is wrong or bad about the person, rather than on strengths and what is going well. Self-talk perpetuates the feeling of shame by keeping the inner dialogue focused on 'I *am* bad and unworthy', which goes to a deeper place than guilt, which is 'I *did* bad.'

With Addiction, it may be impossible to know what thoughts are fed by the diseased part of the brain and which are fed by the rational, recovery part of the self. The diseased brain can be very tricky and can make the person in recovery believe the negative statements. This is why it is impossible to do recovery on one's own, as other people are necessary for checking out thoughts and perceptions that at times may be inaccurate and fuelled by disease. Having a support network of people who understand Addiction and recovery concepts and who can provide honest feedback about what they are hearing is an essential tool for recovery growth, including in the area of self-talk. Often the diseased mind will take you for a ride and convince you of the legitimacy of your own plans. Unfortunately, this is what Addiction does and it can lead to devastating consequences, including relapse. Therefore, having supports where you can test out your thoughts and perceptions is an important part of the self-talk journey.

Receiving feedback on how much you are living in your thinking is also important, as Addiction has a tendency to intellectualize everything and avoid feelings. When exploring self-talk, it is important to look at the feelings that are being generated by your internal dialogue. Feelings are the best guide to telling you if you are in disease territory or recovery, so having regular check-ins with the self about feelings is a useful daily recovery tool.

At this point, you may be confused about what self-talk is, and how to change it in a healthy way. That is okay. You may not be ready to explore this. If you are curious about how to move forward with self-talk, then it will be important for you to read the next section. If you do not feel ready, that is okay. These tools and resources will always be at your disposal when you need them and are ready. Take the recovery journey at your own pace and stay in the process.

Practicing healthy self-talk, or shifting self-talk in a healthy direction, is both simple and complex. The complexity comes from the overwhelming number of thoughts people have in a day, which all come with associated feelings and, at times, behaviours. The simplicity is in the tool: your thoughts are yours alone, and only you have access to them. If you listen, get support, and practice, then shifting self-talk is possible.

In a nutshell, the process of dealing with self-talk is to gain awareness of thoughts; connect with the feelings generated by these thoughts; identify the thoughts that are not serving health or recovery; develop healthy alternatives to the common self-defeating thoughts; and practice catching and challenging your thinking and implementing the healthy alternatives over time.

Journaling or writing down the thoughts is the most straightforward way to develop clarity and awareness around your thinking. This involves either taking time throughout the day, or once a day if your schedule does not permit more frequent journaling, to ask yourself, 'What have I been thinking about today?' You can also ask, 'What are the situations that I have encountered and what have the resulting thoughts been?'

It is important to be specific with the language and connect with the exact words that you use to describe yourself or a situation. For example, 'I am such an idiot,' 'What is wrong with me?', or 'This is totally useless and will not get me anywhere.' This supports the other steps of identifying and shifting self-talk because it gives you concrete examples to work with and a specific idea of how your thinking is supporting or detracting from recovery. This step will likely take a few weeks to gain a solid footing in, as it is important to allow yourself to encounter various situations and challenges to see how your thinking responds. Keep a daily journal or write down thoughts as you notice them. You may begin to see patterns or it may seem like a random mixture of thoughts. Either is acceptable, the important part is to be connected to your inner dialogue and tune into the 'radio' rather than coasting on autopilot and not paying attention.

When journaling your situations and thoughts to gain awareness, it is also important to connect with the associated feelings. For instance, when thinking 'I am such an idiot,' you may notice that you feel frustrated at the same time. After being turned down for a promotion and thinking 'what is wrong with me?' the resultant feelings may be rejection, disappointment, anger, and sadness. There is no right or wrong when it comes to journaling thoughts and feelings; this is our internal perspective. Identifying and validating the feelings, rather than judging, censoring, or avoiding them, help build self-esteem as you begin to support the idea that 'I am worth it and my feelings are worthy too.' Feelings can come in varying degrees and may seem contradictory (e.g., feeling contentment and frustration at the same time), but all of it is okay.

Once there has been an opportunity to journal thoughts and feelings, it is often easier to identify where change may be needed in self-talk. For example, one may notice a particular phrase or statement that they say to themselves repeatedly, such as, 'Geez, what is wrong with me?' It may not even be the same statement that keeps being repeated, but a similar message, for instance that *I am less than* or *I am not good enough* that comes up in different situations. The emotional impact of this inner dialogue is likely also clearer by this point. Shame, low self-worth, frustration, depression, or anxiety are just a few potential side effects of these thoughts, which in turn can propel behaviours like isolation, increased errors, lack of motivation, or giving up on projects.

Once you have an idea of where change is needed in your inner dialogue, it is important to look at developing alternative statements or phrases that, over time, can come to replace the pessimistic talk that is currently there. This can be challenging and support from others in recovery and professionals may be necessary to support this change, as a particular way of thinking can be so ingrained that thinking outside of the box may feel impossible, although it is not.

Let us go back to Samantha, the example from earlier. Through some journaling and self-awareness, she realized that she beats herself up whenever minor mistakes are made, such as dropping something or misplacing an object. She has identified that her inner dialogue involves such phrases as 'What an idiot you are,' 'Everyone is right about you; you're useless,' and 'Just get it together!' Samantha imagines what she might say to someone she cares about who was saying similar things to themselves. 'Maybe you could be more compassionate,' she begins. 'Say something like, *you misplaced that, but it's okay, mistakes are part of being human.*' Another alternative could be, '*You are frustrated right now but that does not invalidate you as a human. You are worthy and loveable.*' A third alternative could be, '*I accept myself for these minor mistakes and appreciate that these are part of me, but do not define me.*'

Altering internal dialogue involves compassion and acceptance. Some people will use affirmations, which are powerful phrases that carry a great deal of personal meaning. Examples can include, 'I am worthy,' 'I am strong,' and 'My feelings are my feelings and they are okay.' Affirmations can be used to replace self-defeating statements and can also be repeated throughout the day to support a shift towards more compassionate inner dialogue, even in the absence of any disruptive chatter.

When exploring self-talk, people often get frustrated and may say that this tool does not work because they have not noticed a shift in their thinking or subsequent feelings. While this may be the case, often the barrier comes from a lack of routine and practice rather than a deficiency in the tool itself. Common sense would tell us that if our thinking drives feelings and behaviour, shifting it in a direction that is kind, compassionate, and realistic would produce benefits in feeling and action. This is a fact that is hard to argue against. The pitfall is that our thinking may be so entrenched, especially when Addiction is present, that vigilance, time, attention, and lots of practice is necessary to move us in that direction. Therefore, once you have decided to explore your self-talk, it important to build this into your daily self-care routine and create reminders for yourself to journal, practice affirmations, write out situation-thoughts-feelings, and whatever other action you are interested in following through on. Daily practice and attention will need to be paid to your thinking for at least one month until the habit starts to become more natural. This does not mean the process ends or finishes after one month, but at this time, the tools you have been using to address your self-talk will be routine and require less overt energy and time. The work, however, will continue, as in recovery and life.

CHAPTER SUMMARY

Distortion in thinking, also known as addictive thinking, is not unique to Addiction, and all of us can be challenged by cognitive distortions. This typically occurs when we feel insecure, have low self-esteem, feel stressed, and have difficulty adjusting to life's challenges. Addictive thinking does not necessarily indicate Addiction, but the intensity and regularity of this type of thinking is most common among people with the disease. Addictive thoughts are irrational and can manifest in a number of psychological strategies, including all-or-nothing thinking, rationalization, and denial. Addictive thinking propagates feelings of guilt and shame in the person experiencing them.

Addictive thinking generally precedes the use of substances or addictive behaviours and precipitates relapse in people with Addiction. Holistic recovery is a framework for developing awareness of addictive thinking and lessening the impact it has on daily living. A goal of treatment with all addictive thinking is to increase awareness of distorted perceptions, talk about the feelings, and take recovery action. Awareness alone is not enough and the commitment to recovery action in turn creates more awareness and the change necessary to grow.

Increased self-awareness occurs by talking and getting feedback from those you trust, as everyone has blind spots that they may be unable to see or hear—but others can. The Johari Window, a technique used in counselling, helps increase self-awareness and allows people to better understand their relationship with themselves and others. Self-talk is another valuable tool for health and wellness development, a term used to refer to the ongoing, internal conversation that people have with themselves and is beneficial to explore as part of recovery from Addiction. Developing awareness and practicing healthy self-talk can lead to benefits in many areas, including dealing with stress more effectively, exploring feelings honestly, and improving self-worth and esteem. Journaling is a very important tool to become aware of one's self-talk and feedback from others is essential to ensure awareness of healthy recovery thoughts and the disease-related distortions. More information on how to journal can be found in Appendix B.

Chapter 4: Addictive Feeling

In this chapter, we distinguish between feelings and emotions. We explore in depth the common emotions and feelings present in active Addiction to gain more awareness about them and learn how to process them in a healthy way. We learn that feelings are not bad or good, though one may want good ones and to avoid bad ones. Rather, they are useful sources of information to guide behaviours, consciously or subconsciously.

Addiction is about escape, relief, and reward, generally from feelings. This is the reason that both celebratory feelings and painful, difficult, or uncomfortable feelings can increase vulnerability for people with Addiction. The idea that there is no such thing as a bad feeling, even if it feels bad, can initially seem ludicrous to people with Addiction because, when the disease is present, *all* feelings are overwhelming and may appear bad. They are something to be numbed, made to go away, and pushed aside. In the short and long run, however, avoidance of feelings only exacerbates the disease and fuels its progression.

FEELINGS AND EMOTIONS

There can be a great deal of confusion between feelings and emotions. Some people and health care providers use them synonymously, whereas others distinguish carefully between the two. Historically, the word feeling was meant to connote anything that could be taken in or experienced via the five senses of sound, sight, touch, taste, and smell. These are your feelings. Emotion has often been used to refer to our subjective, inner experience and associated with words such as fear, grief, shame, happiness, joy, contentment, anger, and rage. The American Psychological Association's (APA) *Dictionary of Psychology* states that the word feeling[1] is reserved for the conscious, subjective experience of emotion that is an internal response to internal or external stimuli. Simply put, this means that the feelings are being realized, or felt, by the individual, whereas emotion results from an internal physiological response that is elicited by something happening inside the individual or some external stressors or events.

Emotions are constantly being generated throughout the day while one is alone or interacting with others. Every interaction, thought, experience, and activity comes with an emotional response, whether you are aware of it at the feelings level or not. Emotions can be conscious or unconscious and emoting is just an expression of the emotions through feelings, which can be dramatic with the disease taking over or therapeutic as honesty takes hold.

Avoidance of expressing feelings happens because of the disease of Addiction. When someone is actively seeking to become numb, the emotional constipation grows to the point where an overflow, or release, happens. This can be subtle, where a person hides from others, or dramatic such as suicide attempts, self-harm, rage, or uncontrollable crying. While the individual may feel like these episodes came out of nowhere, they usually have been building for days, weeks, months, or even years. All of the unprocessed and unrealized emotions eventually catch up with the individual and come out as painful, or what can feel like unmanageable, feelings. It is essential that emotions be moved from the unconscious to the conscious level for healthy recovery, or else this periodic constipation and overflowing will continue to happen, causing the phenomenon of the 'dry drunk'[2] as talked about in 12- step circles. This is the notion that someone is abstinent from their substance(s) of choice, but still experiencing the dysfunctional emotional response characteristic of Addiction, which makes them appear intoxicated as their thoughts, feelings, and behaviours seem the same as when they had been using. They struggle to become aware of emotions, feel them, and process them in a healthy manner.

Initially it may seem difficult to move emotions from an unconscious level to a conscious, feelings level. It certainly can be, particularly if years and plenty of practice have gone into avoiding, numbing, and stuffing them. The main ways to move emotions into awareness are:

- Journaling (Appendix B)

- Learn about the various feelings out there (e.g., have a feelings list that you can refer to as you develop your vocabulary, such as that found in Appendix C)

- Talk to healthy supports, especially other people in recovery, as this can help you gain clarity on what you are feeling

- Spend time each day asking 'How am I feeling?'

- Meditation

Throughout the rest of this chapter, we explore topics related to the common feelings that are present in active Addiction and can flare up in the early days of recovery. It is important to note that these feelings are not limited to people in active Addiction and early recovery, but are present for everyone. However, the consequences of not exploring them for people with Addiction are more severe, as in the worst case scenario, the unaddressed feelings can lead to behavioural relapse.

FEELINGS IN ADDICTION

Guilt and shame.[3] Confusion abounds when it comes to the feelings of guilt and shame. Much like with feelings and emotions, many people use the terms synonymously. Others believe that it is critical to distinguish between guilt and shame for recovery and that it can also be helpful to distinguish them from other feelings, like humiliation and embarrassment.

Humiliation involves degradation, can be related to our social status, and often involves other people. Humiliation does not feel deserved, like when you spill something on your shirt at a social gathering and everyone laughs. Embarrassment involves intense discomfort with oneself and is often experienced when a socially unacceptable act is witnessed by or revealed to others. For example, you forget to wash your hands after leaving the restroom and a colleague reveals that to your boss. People can live with humiliation and embarrassment, as they are often short-lived and fleeting feelings, though uncomfortable.

Guilt is the feeling that occurs when a person believes that they have violated a moral standard that they themselves believe in. It lives at the level of thinking, as the person will reflect on the action that led them to guilt. For example, someone may feel guilty about not sending a birthday card to their parent, or calling their partner a jackass during an argument. They may spend days or weeks playing over the situation in their head and trying to identify what they could have done differently to prevent it from happening. Guilt is, in sum, 'I did bad.'

Shame is the emotion related to the feeling of 'I am bad.' It is an intensely painful and uncomfortable emotion. It can be devastating and perpetual. When people feel shame, they feel unworthy. Whereas humiliation does not feel deserved, shame does. 'You deserve to have people laugh at you because you are an idiot.' 'You should be fired because you are incompetent, you loser.' 'I cannot tell anyone that I have Addiction or else I will be blacklisted.' These are just a few examples of shame-based thinking. Shame often involves events that no one has ever witnessed, and tends to thrive in secrecy. For instance, Addictive behaviours and the lying involved in sneaking, hiding, and manipulating make great fodder for shame. These are things that are uncharacteristic and seem too dangerous to reveal to anybody else because of what it would say about you. What would people think if they knew you hid bottles of vodka in the laundry room? That you could not attend your grandmother's 80th birthday party because you were high? That you sneak into the kitchen and eat chocolate chips from the baking cupboard because you have emptied the house of all other binge food?

Shame is a core emotion and generates the deepest feelings that people can experience. It reflects our sense of self and impacts confidence, esteem, and worth. People can experience shame in a variety of areas of our lives, including with age, appearance, roles (as parents, employees, children, etc.), money, status, and health. Shame is often connected to expectations that you carry or perceive are being placed on you by people around you. For instance, 'You should have X number of dollars in your bank account to be successful' is an expectation that people may carry. When people do not live up to that standard, the resulting feeling is shame. The sad thing with shame is that, until the feeling itself is recognized and processed, even if you had X number of dollars in the bank, the feeling of shame would persist because, ultimately, self-worth and confidence cannot be tied to external factors like wealth, power, or status. If shame is present then you will be perpetually pursuing an elusive ideal. Money or the accolades of others will not make you happy, only you will.

The antidote to shame is serenity, which means appreciating and being comfortable with yourself *as you are*. You can still have goals and aspirations but these do not have to be met to feel worthy. Serenity says, 'I am okay as I am today.' It is also important to let go of the shoulds, or expectations that people carry of themselves and others, for both of these things keep you trapped in looking for external solutions to internal issues. Anytime you are 'shoulding' on yourself, you are heaping on more shame. For example, 'I should have run that race faster' invalidates the fact that you finished your first competitive race and feeds into your shameful belief that you are a loser.

Within our physical body, shame resides in the solar plexus chakra,[4] which is the third chakra in energy healing (see Appendix

F for more information on this topic). It is located between the rib cage and navel region and is associated with many core parts of self, including identity, self-confidence, worth, purpose, and relationships. It is important to understand that when people are out of balance in any of the energy centres, or chakras, people run at either a higher or lower level of energy. This means that they do not feel balanced or in equilibrium internally. Things like stress, conflict, and disease can disrupt our internal balance and cause people to run energetically high or low.

When the energy in your solar plexus chakra runs high, people notice they become aggressive, project superiority and ego, are overpowering, forceful, quarrelsome, threatening, pushy, intense, rebellious, power-loving, competitive, hyped up, ruthless, workaholic, disconnected, angry, lack tolerance, and fear intimacy. Many of these traits describe what is commonly known as the 'type A personality'[3]. This personality is usually associated with high levels of shame and lack of confidence that people are trying to compensate for by a focus on overdoing and achievement.

When the energy in the solar plexus chakra runs low, people notice a number of symptoms including that they feel fragile, lack determination and intention, have negative internal dialogue, lack confidence, feel inferior, have low self-worth, limited courage, feel an inner void, and are lonely. They may also notice that they suck energy from other people by being dependent or needy and may have a lot of phobias or fears. While this person may present a lot differently than the type A individual, at core they are both coming from the same place: a reaction to high amounts of shame and low levels of self-worth. 'If only they knew the real me' is the fear that comes with both a high amount of ego and low amount of confidence, but both are fundamentally from the same root of shame.

People who carry a lot of shame will often describe digestive issues (stomach upset, nausea, and diarrhea) as well as tightness in the chest or stomach. Common physical ailments related to shame include ulcers, panic attacks, diabetes, eating disorders, insomnia, confusion, fatigue, stress, and Addiction. When people are balanced, they find they have success in their professional and personal life, are more spontaneous and flexible, are self-confident, and have healthy relationships with others.

It can be a gradual process to move from shame to serenity and into self-worth and acceptance, but it is also the most gratifying part of recovery. This is because, ultimately, it brings you closer to you. To start moving from shame to serenity:

a. Become more aware of how shame manifests in your thinking, feeling, and body. How do you think when you are shameful? What is the internal dialogue? Where do you feel shame in your body? What are the consequences of shame to you, behaviourally and emotionally?

b. Be honest. Talk about your feeling of shame wherever and whenever you can. The more shame is released, the less powerful it becomes.

c. Journal. This is another helpful release for the feeling of shame, even if you are not sure what situation it may be tied to. Refer to Appendix B for information on how to journal

d. Try new activities. Being surrounded by different people and new activities helps give clarity on self, which increases acceptance and diminishes shame.

For those in active Addiction and early recovery, the lines between guilt and shame can seem blurred. Usually people are carrying a lot of guilt for actions taken during their disease, which makes it easy to lose sight of the deeper, underlying emotion of shame. It is critical that shame be talked about because it is the secrets that keep us sick. Addiction feeds on shame, as it wants people to believe they are useless, unworthy, and deserving of pain and suffering. This way the Addiction is more likely to get what it wants: instant gratification and relief through acting out behaviour. Shame is also strongly tied to another core emotion—fear.

Fear. The connection between shame and fear can be elusive at first, but as you begin to familiarize yourself with these related feelings, the connection becomes obvious. Let us start by exploring and defining it. Fear is another core emotion that reflects our biological response to perceived physical or emotional threats. It helps protect us when there is danger, but can also exist when the threat is only imagined. This is where fear can be unhealthy and lead to long-term health issues, as the body is living in a chronic state of distress and preparation for action or flight. Imagined fears become just as real to the body as if you were being chased by a bear so, similarly to stress, certain systems like your gastrointestinal and digestive systems slow down so that you are ready to fight or escape as needed. The problem is, because the threat is often imaginary, there is no start or end point so the body can live in this state for much longer than intended, whether that be hours, days, weeks, or months. This creates a lot of wear and tear to the physical self, and erodes people emotionally. Most of what is feared in the imagination is unlikely to come to fruition, so a lot of internal energy and resources are depleted by thinking about them. Fear has the mind living in the future, which fuels anxiety and adds to the perceived distress, although none of it is based in reality. This process occurs for everyone, but it is heightened with the catastrophic thinking that comes with Addiction, as discussed in Chapter 3.

Fear can stand for *False Evidence Appearing Real*. Staying present and focusing on the here and now is required to reduce fear, but with addictive thinking, the mind takes a person to days, weeks, and months ahead. It is important to become consciously aware of when one's thoughts are caught up in fortune telling or writing a script for the future without any supporting evidence in an effort to reduce morbid expectations and fear.

You may be starting to see that fear feeds off shame, and vice versa. If people feel less than, as shame would have you believe, then there can be many things in life to create fear. For example, the biggest fear is that of being real. 'What will people think when they know the real me?' Shame tells you that you are unlikeable. Therefore, people will judge, reject, or abandon us if the mask comes off and the authentic self is revealed. This fear can lead people to be inauthentic; to live according to an external script they have created from society. This theoretically prevents this rejection from occurring. This fuels shame because people start to believe this is the only acceptable self and anything less than is unworthy. Who can live up to an ideal script? No one. When caught in this predicament, the behavioural response of wanting to control the outcome surfaces, as well as anger and a myriad of associated feelings.

Control related to fear and shame. With Addiction, shame from the past and fear of the future are predominant emotions that generate numerous feelings, which lead to increased desire for control. Shame keeps people stuck and unable to live in the moment because they are preoccupied with events from the past. With shame as the predominant emotion, the person tries to control their world in an effort to reduce it, but it is both unproductive and counterproductive.

Case History: Bev. *Bev decided to break up with Dan after six months because she didn't feel like he was meeting her needs. She felt hurt and angry that he wasn't more considerate of her feelings, so she became increasingly irritated and angry with him in the hope that he would clue into her feelings. Bev grew up in an abusive home where the consistent message from her parents was that she was demanding, needy, and difficult to love. Her relationship with Dan was triggering many painful memories from her childhood. Bev believed that to keep from being hurt, she would try to control her feelings of inadequacy and vulnerability, and had been selective about revealing her true self to Dan. After six months, this was not working for her anymore and Bev's need to be in charge and have things her way was creating a wedge in their relationship. It made Dan more distant, despite the fact that she was working hard to take care of his needs. Bev was able to justify and explain her motives for breaking* *up with him and give reasons for her controlling behaviour, but this didn't help her get what she wanted, which was Dan's love and affection.*

Bev's story is not uncommon, as it demonstrates how easy and subtle it is to move from a place of fear and shame to control. Unfortunately, it also emphasizes the reality that control does not lessen fear or shame, but drives them to become further entrenched. Ultimately, the controlling behaviours reinforce the fear and shame as they create barriers in relationships and with self.

As we have discussed, fear is an emotion induced by a perceived threat, typically a future event that has yet to occur. It is a basic survival mechanism occurring in response to a specific stimulus, such as pain or the threat of danger. In short, fear is the ability to recognize danger, leading to an urge to confront it or flee from it, also known as the fight-or-flight response. When people feel fear, typical behaviours include escape and avoidance. Fear can also be an instant reaction to something presently happening and all people have an instinctual response to potential danger, which is in fact important for survival. However, when fear is based on distorted perceptions of threats and danger, it can become maladaptive. Maladaptive behaviour often follows in an attempt to reduce one's anxiety, but the result is dysfunctional and non-productive in alleviating the actual problem and becomes counter-productive in the long-term. You get more of what you are trying to control or avoid.

Letting go of control means allowing ourselves to be supported and trusting that things will turn out as they are meant to, even if that is not how you had envisioned. It is not always easy, although it can be. As you practice and expand your capacity to let go, you are then able to release and transform a large amount of unnecessary stress, worry, and anxiety from your life, work, and relationships. There are many things you can do to let go of control. It is important to remember that this is a process and something that may not come easily. Many of us have been trained, directly or indirectly, to be controlling. In certain situations at work or home, being controlling has been encouraged or seemed necessary for our own survival and of those around us. That being said, if you have realized your controlling behaviour is not serving you well, here are some things you can do to let go:

a. Be honest with yourself about your own controlling nature. It probably varies a bit for you, as it does for everyone, but at the same time everyone has certain tendencies, especially in the most important and stressful areas of our lives. Take a look at where, how, and why you hold on to control. Be honest with yourself about what this costs and how it affects you and those around you.

b. Look at whether you are willing to let go of control. This is an important question to ponder and to answer honestly. In some cases, the answer may be no. It is important to honour that if that is the case for you. The more willing you are to ask and answer this question, the more likely you are to start letting go of control consciously if the answer is yes. You may not know how to do it or what it would look like, but authentic willingness is always the first step to positive change.

c. Consider who could support you. Getting support is one of the most important, and often most vulnerable, aspects of letting go of control. Even though you may feel like you are alone, that no one gets it, or that you could not possibly ask for help, the reality is that it is difficult to let go of control without the support of other people. The irony of asking for help is that many of us do not feel comfortable doing so and worry that it makes us seem weak or needy. On the other side, most of us love to be asked for help and really enjoy helping others. Remember that you cannot do it alone. The good news is that most of us have many people in our life that would jump at the chance to support us, if you were willing to ask for help more freely.

d. Surrender. This is the bottom line of letting go. Surrendering does not mean giving up or not caring, it means trusting and allowing things to be taken care of by others, by the process and by the inexplicable forces of physics, chemistry, and biology governing life. Some call this force universal intelligence, some call it God, some spirit, some nature, and some do not call it anything, but most of us have an experience of it at some level. Surrendering is about consciously choosing to trust whatever makes sense to us beyond ourselves and have faith in the process without attachment to making things happen. It is something that can liberate us in a profound way and is all about us choosing to let go. This is different from avoidance and pretending to let go when you may not even have faced what you need to honestly. For some people, faith means religion. We mean faith as acceptance of life on life's terms. Religion may be the vehicle of faith in some instances, or not. Our experience has demonstrated to us that faith is the antidote to fear.

When you look back on your life, you usually see that things happened for a reason. What if you lived in the present moment with this same hindsight awareness? As a mentor said to one of us years ago, 'You are living your life as though you are trying to survive it. You have to remember, no one ever has.' Another emotional cost to wanting to control the outcome and living in fear, shame, and guilt is anger.

Anger. As with the other core emotions we have covered (shame and fear), there is a lot of misunderstanding about anger. At its root, anger is the response to expectations not matching reality, which, like fear, has evolutionary advantages. It can offer protection and motivates us to change things that appear to be threats, especially when they happen unexpectedly. Today, however, the threats to our wellbeing are less straightforward; they are often created by our mind rather than the reality of a situation. Rather than anger being our response to one situation in which you felt threatened, it is often an amalgamation of responses to a variety of situations.

Let us explore this idea further. Reflect on when you tend to get angry about. Is it when there is a life threatening situation or is it usually a reaction to daily stressors? For most, anger is often over the silliest things, like someone leaving dishes in the sink, cutting you off in traffic, or making a snide remark. You are not alone if you identify that your anger flares up at the most unexpected times. This is because people go through a variety of seemingly harmless and non-threatening situations throughout the day, such as waiting in line. Dealing with these life problems, including children's temper tantrums or seeing our partners grumpy, can all generate feelings of irritability and frustration that, left unchecked, can build to anger. Often the mind will focus on the mundane while ignoring something deeper that you are truly unhappy with such as dissatisfaction with work, a spouse, or not having enough self-care time. If you continue to focus on surface situations and not address more fundamental issues, the real feelings become repressed or suppressed. Then, usually at the most inopportune times, there is a proverbial straw to break the camel's back that sends all of the emotional responses (feelings) you have been ignoring into overflow, not unlike a backup with a pipe that has become clogged over time.

This overflow may come out as outbursts such as yelling, physical aggression, swearing, name calling or the like, but underneath are a variety of feelings. These may include, but are not limited to, frustration, irritation, hurtfulness, and feeling overwhelmed or out of control. Feeling manipulated or controlled can evoke strong feelings related to the emotion of anger, especially when you feel that you are not being heard or feel that you are being duped. Jealousy and envy, which are more shame-related, can come out as anger. As you can imagine, the powerful feelings that people carry but are avoiding percolate in the subconscious until they can no longer be avoided. The resulting emotion is anger, but that is the tip of the feelings iceberg. What is underneath the surface is less visible, which are the other feelings you have been carrying but ignoring. These feelings are what need to be explored honestly for healthy recovery to be possible. Living on the surface and dealing with just the anger usually has limited benefit. Deep breathing, taking time outs, counting from one to ten, and channeling this energy into physical output (i.e., exercise) do not ultimately get at the core of the anger, which often contains fear, shame, and guilt, in addition to a whole variety of other uncomfortable feelings. If you are honest with yourself and others about the feelings that are being generated by your past, present, and future, this will be the key to letting go of anger and living in peace, serenity, and surrender. Moving from the addictive emotion of anger to healthy recovery involves:

a. Honesty with your feelings to yourself.

b. Asking yourself 'what is this anger about?' as well as 'what other feelings may be tied to my anger?'

c. Keeping yourself and others safe. Give yourself a safe, calm, quiet place to relax to allow the intensity of your anger to lessen before communicating with others and exploring the feeling further for yourself.

Doing this emotional work requires humility, the need to ask for help, and looking honestly at things you may not be happy about, which can interfere with the innate defense mechanism of shame–pride.

Pride[5] **and Grandiosity.**[6] As with many feelings in the context of Addiction, pride and grandiosity are connected to shame and can flare up during active disease when minimization and denial are high. Although pride is often talked about as a desirable feeling in oneself related to achievement by ourselves or by others you feel connected to, it can become an inflated sense of self, status, or accomplishments. Grandiosity refers to a sense of superiority to others, where the inflated sense of self becomes a way of life, disconnected with reality. Other words used synonymously with pride and grandiosity include ego, vanity, and hubris—all variations on the theme of an inflated, unrealistic sense of self.

Do not get fooled into thinking pride and grandiosity are evidence of self-worth, because the key commonality with both feelings is that they are artificial, meaning that they are not connected to reality, either externally or internally. These disconnections happen when people start comparing themselves to other people. Even though you will never know the full reality of your own or other people's inner worlds, you end up comparing your insides to other people's outsides, which may also be coloured with distortions. This comparison will always be imbalanced and inaccurate. What you see in others, or the image that people put forth of themselves, can never capture the full reality of that individual.

If you end up comparing your external image (e.g., money, power, status, profession) to other people's external image, which happens automatically when pride or grandiosity are activated, it is superficial at best. Pride and grandiosity are used as a cover to the true feeling of shame, which one can also call inferiority, insecurity, self-doubt, or lack of self-worth that one truly feels within. Pride and grandiosity are all about image management; doing, saying, or being anything to fit in, look successful, popular, funny, witty, charming, powerful, smart, strong, or whatever characteristics the mind believes are necessary to be accepted by others. The connection to shame is that while people are trying to impress the world, they are losing sight of themselves and may start to believe that who they truly are is not good enough because they can never live up to the unrealistic standards set by self, but driven by others and society. The result is trying even harder to fit in or act as if they are successful, which feeds pride, grandiosity and, ultimately, Addiction. The following image depicts the vicious cycle that these feelings can put people in.

Shame $\longleftrightarrow$ Pride/Grandiosity $\longleftrightarrow$ Act "as if"

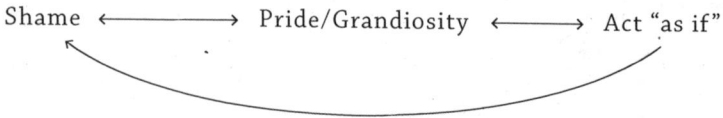

FIGURE 2 CYCLE OF SHAME AND PRIDE

There is a lot of denial around pride and grandiosity. The individual living in this mind-state has a difficult time seeing that they are not living authentically or honestly. This is not to say that this is a conscious process; more often than not, it is the addicted mind driving this denial so that it seems natural, comfortable, and familiar, and is operating at a subconscious level of being. Ultimately, however, living in pride and grandiosity keeps people stuck, trapped in a land of superficialities, unrealistic standards, and constant judgment. This provides no understanding of what is happening within, which is often too painful or difficult for people to look at, especially when Addiction has them in its throes. Once the veil of denial is lifted, people are left to face the deep-seated feeling of shame and have to look honestly at the question of 'who am I?' There is tremendous opportunity in this process, but it can be hard to see during active Addiction and in the early days of recovery, when feelings are strong but coping strategies are underdeveloped.

Do you experience moments in which you feel prideful or grandiose but other times where you feel a lot of self-hatred or self-loathing? This is another common consequence of living with Addiction. The experiences of shame, pride, and grandiosity are not usually separate and come from the same root of not knowing, liking, or accepting one's self. It is not surprising that the inner experience can oscillate from one to the other, sometimes slowly and sometimes quickly, depending on the individual. This can feed into the Jekyll and Hyde phenomenon that many people observe in themselves or others with Addiction. A person feels moments of ego, determination, stubbornness, or will when pride and grandiosity are active, and at other times experiences extreme isolation, self-harm, and self-hate when shame has taken over. The shame is often driven by the comparison of one's insides with other people's outsides, which appear well put together.

The key to moving from addictive feeling to recovery when it comes to this vicious cycle of shame, pride, and grandiosity is to:

a. Stop acting to please others or to get strokes from others. Ask yourself regularly, 'What is my motivation for doing or saying this?' and, 'How am I feeling right now?' If you feel uncomfortable or distressed, chances are that you are going against your natural internal needs.

Change your course of action. This may require pulling back from people, events, or activities to gain clarity on whether they are healthy for you or not.

a. Use affirmations and gratitude to begin building self-acceptance and serenity.

Take time daily to reflect on feelings and ask yourself 'What do I need?' This will help prevent you from becoming caught up in thinking about what others expect of you.

The feelings discussed thus far are not independent. Getting more honest with one feeling, such as pride or grandiosity, can bring to the surface other feelings, such as fear of judgment, in which people worry about how others view them and what they think. In this context, fear can be directly related to fear of rejection or abandonment.

Rejection and abandonment. Addiction is a family disease and, even if parents or caregivers did not have an obvious manifestation of it, chances are that it has affected them at some level. Therefore, many people with Addiction have been raised in households in which parenting discipline, affection, boundaries, or communication was limited or inconsistent. This can create vulnerability to feeling rejected or abandoned. Where people are raised lays the groundwork for safety and attachment. If this is not present, for whatever reason, it can lay an unstable framework for the growing child. During active Addiction, people who were raised in homes where there was a lot of chaos, lack of family time, lack of discussion about feelings, and neglect of care or responsibility may notice their sensitivity to feelings of rejection or abandonment being triggered. Many people have also experienced loss of a parent in their childhood through death or divorce. Not knowing a father, or being raised by a single mother or by another relative creates many feelings that can be difficult to talk about. The reactionary response may be to become clingy and dependent on other people, or to isolate and pull away from others because this feels safer. The dysfunctional emotional response (E) characteristic of Addiction can create a skewed perception of reality, leading one to interpret others' words or actions through the lens of rejection or abandonment when this may not be the case. This perpetuates problems in relationships and fuels disease activity to become numb or escape from these uncomfortable experiences.

Underneath this fear or feeling of rejection or abandonment resides shame, the other addiction-related emotion. How are all of these experiences and feelings connected? If you are already carrying a high level of shame, you likely do not feel worthy of the relationships or opportunities in your life, which creates an undercurrent of fear. What will happen when they discover the real me? The answer that the addicted mind scripts is that these people will leave when they discover the real you because that person is inherently unlovable. This, of course, is a fantasy and rarely happens in reality, but the thoughts and feelings in Addiction are very powerful and convince people that this is the guaranteed outcome. This can then lead to the person putting on a mask and pretending to be someone they are not in the hopes that people will deem them good enough and not leave.

The ironic reality is that if this situation truly did happen, meaning that someone rejected you for being yourself, it would provide you valuable information about them and your relationship. It can reveal dysfunction that you may have overlooked. You do not need someone in your life who cannot handle the real you. This is something that the mind of the person with Addiction can have a hard time comprehending and accepting. Instead, it fights and says, 'No, this only speaks to my weaknesses and failures, it does not say anything about the other person.' Addiction thrives on distress, shame, and degradation, and will play tricks on the mind to fuel this.

To work on self-acceptance one can:

a. Take an honest look at existing relationships and consider, 'Does that person contribute to my recovery?' To understand this, ask yourself, 'How do I feel when I am around that person?' If there is discomfort, awkwardness, or image management, these are clues that this is not a healthy relationship for you.

b. Practice spending time on your own. Fear of rejection becomes strongest when the mind is convinced that you need specific people to survive. If you build up comfort being yourself, than interactions with others become a joy and not filled with fear and anxiety.

c. Be honest about your feelings of fear, rejection, or abandonment as they arise with healthy supports or through journaling. Any time you expose your feelings, the power they have to create problems within you lessens.

If people do not deal with their fear of rejection and avoid their feelings, needs, and preferences, over time this can lead to strong feelings of resentment.

Resentment. Resentment is a deadly poison. It kills anything put in its path if not addressed. It places a wedge between one's relationship with self and the external world. People carry resentments whenever they feel they have been wronged, whether this is real, perceived, or imagined. The intensity and depth of the resentments grows when people feel they have been wronged by someone close to them, or someone in a position of authority or power. This shakes the foundation of trust. More often than not, resentments are kept quiet and become secrets. Even when resentments are not being expressed, they tend to come out in other ways, such as physical ailments (ulcers, skin rashes, etc.); short-temperedness or irritability; an increased desire to escape or numb through substances or behaviours; and increased bitterness, anger, or isolation.

As with all other feelings, resentments cannot be avoided or escaped from indefinitely. While resentments are often directed outwards (e.g., 'I resent my father for leaving when I was twelve'), people can also carry resentment towards ourselves. This type of resentment is usually the strongest and hardest to look at. One may resent oneself for staying in an unhealthy relationship, continuing to use drugs and alcohol despite destructive consequences, and the list goes on. Anytime you carry high standards for yourself and others, you are planting the seeds for future resentments.

This means people need to let go of expectations to prevent resentments from forming. This brings up many questions. Namely, if you do not have expectations, how will you achieve anything? People need goals to move forward in life but these are different from expectations. The table below outlines the differences between expectations and goals.

Table 1. The Difference Between Expectations and Goals

Expectations	Goals
Are rigid	Are flexible
Are based on 'shoulds'	Are based on hopes and aims
Need to happen a certain way	Can unfold as they need to
Are tied to the outcome	Are open to various outcomes
The process to meet them is fixed	The process is fluid and changes as it goes

Expectations	Goals
Lead to disappointment and resentment	Lead to contentment and a feeling of success
Are 'musts'	Are desires

As you can see, expectations are set-in-stone conceptualizations of what outcome needs to happen and the process by which to get there. This can open up the door to resentment at any point in the process, as well as if the expectation is not achieved. For example, you have a friend you are concerned about. They have been complaining about pain in their abdomen for many weeks. If you were living in expectations, you would generate a list of things your friend needed to do in order to get well. If you were living with goals, you would talk openly with your friend about their challenges, roadblocks, and options for getting help and support, rather than being prescriptive about the path forward.

It is easy to develop resentments when you live with expectations. What would happen if your friend did not follow your recommendations, or did them differently than expected? What if they still had pain after following your list? In this scenario, not only were you tied to the process of how your friend should get well, you were also tied to the outcome of them being pain-free at the end. People can trap themselves in expectations very quickly, both with others and ourselves. The same situation could be applied to self. For example, you were having pain and wanted to find relief. Would you choose the path of goals, which means openness, feedback from others, and flexibility, or the rigid path of expectations?

Resentment[8] is built into step four of all 12-step programs: *We made a searching and fearless moral inventory of ourselves.* On the surface, this step is not directly connected to resentment, but a searching and fearless exploration of all resentments is part of step four that your sponsor can help you with. This is a necessary part of step four because resentments cause so much damage to self and others, as mentioned above. Part of this exploration involves getting honest about how much expectation you were carrying and what role you played in the resentment. Addiction feeds off resentment because it is an uncomfortable feeling from which people want to escape. To reinforce recovery from resentment it is important to:

a. Be aware of your behaviour and feelings around people and in certain situations. If you are snappy or uncomfortable then chances are you are carrying resentment towards that person or yourself.

b. Journal daily about your feelings to become more honest with yourself.

c. Work step four through a 12-step program as part of your healing journey. It is best to process resentment with guidance and support.

An example used above to demonstrate the difference between expectations and goals involved the topic of pain. Pain is an experience that can further complicate one's journey of recovery from Addiction.

Pain. Individuals with Addiction are not immune to other conditions or diseases and may have chronic pain, conditions causing acute pain, or injuries from the past that can be aggravated. Our feelings and physical health are directly linked. As people gain in awareness, they realize that feelings will aggravate physical pain, including pain with a known root cause, and physical pain will drive feelings. This does not mean that feelings necessarily cause physical pain or vice versa. What would be more accurate to say is that each experience will magnify pre-existing vulnerabilities. For instance, if you scraped your finger you may notice that the pain is worse towards the end of the day when you are tired. This does not mean that your fatigue caused the pain, but it magnified a sensation that was already there.

Exploring the relationship between feelings and physical pain also does not mean that the underlying condition or injury causing the pain is not real or that it is all in your head. It means that lack of awareness of feelings can exacerbate this vulnerability. The risk of leaving this unchecked is increased pain and frustration for everyone, Addiction or not. There is the heightened risk that when Addiction is involved, the desire for escape or relief will be higher. The individual is not only vulnerable from a physical health and pain perspective, but their Addiction tends to get aggravated in these situations.

Developing emotional health and awareness is critical for management of pain and injury and can be done in the following ways:

a. Create a health and recovery plan that includes lots of self-care and time for rest and recuperation, in addition to daily responsibilities and recovery action. It is essential that our bodies have time to regenerate and heal. It is important that this time be conscious and purposeful rather than crashing on the couch to watch TV just because you feel like it.

b. Have a physical health plan that includes moderate exercise to maintain strength and mobility, as well as increase natural endorphins, the body's 'feel good' chemicals. This plan can also incorporate lots of fruits, vegetables, and water with a balanced diet.

c. Review all of the suggestions made in previous sections of this chapter. They can provide benefit to those struggling with chronic pain.

Addictive thinking is related to addictive feeling. Minimization, a feature of addictive thinking discussed in Chapter 3, is described below as connected to feelings, as well as the other extreme of exaggeration.

Minimization and exaggeration. The tendency to minimize or exaggerate situations and feelings is a consequence of addictive thinking. This is related to all-or-nothing thinking and catastroph-izing, which are characteristic of people with Addiction. This is the dysfunctional emotional response. Addiction is a disease of escape, relief, and reward, and when feelings are generated, the faulty part of the brain either wants to minimize this (make a molehill out of a mountain) or exaggerate it (make a mountain out of a molehill). This fuels Addiction because either way, it increases unpleasant feel-ings within. By ignoring certain events or feelings, this contributes to emotional constipation, resulting in a tidal wave of feeling down the road, which is incredibly uncomfortable and often drives a desire for escape or relief. In the case of exaggeration, everyday stressors or events become unbearable, unmanageable, and impossible to deal with. This is the challenge of Addiction: to bring emotions into awareness, recognize them, feel the feelings, and process them fairly and realistically without being caught in the traps that Addiction will lay.

CHAPTER SUMMARY

Feelings drive the behaviours that fuel Addiction. Therefore, it is necessary for people in recovery to gain awareness of their feelings and deal with them as they arise, not resort to escaping, numbing, and avoiding, as that is what fed into the sickness to begin with. Addiction feeds on the feelings described in this chapter, because the more unpleasant and uncomfortable you are, the more likely your Addiction is to get the hit it is looking for. Avoidance keeps you in the trap of escape and, thus, not dealing with reality. While the feel-ings may be difficult to experience, this is ultimately what one needs to do in order to get better. Shame, anger, and fear are core emotions that are often at the root of countless feelings. They generate a lot of feelings that lead to control and hiding, even when it would be more prudent to acknowledge what is happening. Any struggles that give rise to more feelings need to be talked about openly and honestly. The more connected you can become, the easier it will be to shine a light on them, which shrinks their power within you and allows you to move further away from the disease and appreciate the joys of recovery.

Chapter 5: Addictive Behaviour

This chapter explores the impact of specific substances and behaviours in Addiction and recovery. Problems related to intoxication, withdrawal, and common medical complications are discussed. We also examine patterns in relationships and what role they play in Addiction. Environment, exposure, and stress are discussed as they are major pathways to relapse. We also explain the Karpman Drama Triangle, sometimes called the Drama Triangle, as it effectively describes the dysfunctional roles individuals may take in relationships. We discuss how transformation to healthier perspectives can happen.

UNDERSTANDING THE IMPACT OF ALCOHOL, DRUGS, AND BEHAVIOURS IN ADDICTION AND RECOVERY, AND THE ROLE OF PRESCRIPTION MEDICATIONS

We will now explore how different substances affect the body and brain, with subsequent impact on thinking, feeling, and behaviour. To appreciate the extent of the impact, it is important to know the chemical nature of substances and how they are classified in terms of how they affect the brain. Substances that are commonly used recreationally by people with or without Addiction can be grouped into four categories: stimulants, depressants, hallucinogens, and organic solvents.

Stimulants include nicotine, caffeine, amphetamines, and cocaine. They usually act directly on specific receptors or can increase the quantity of excitatory neurotransmitters such as norepinephrine or dopamine in the synapses. The synapses are the points of contact between nerve cells to transmit chemical and electrical signals that are essential for optimum brain function.

Depressants include alcohol, benzodiazepines, z-drugs (such as zopiclone), and barbiturates. Alcohol disrupts the function of the brain more diffusely and produces its effects on the reward circuitry through activation of the opioid and cannabinoid neural pathways. Benzodiazepines, z-drugs and barbiturates act more specifically on the GABA receptor complex as an agonist, to amplify the effects of natural compounds that modulate nervous system functioning through the GABA system.

Opioids, such as codeine, morphine, oxycodone, hydromorphone, meperidine, and tramadol, act on the opioid receptors in the brain, which is part of the reward circuitry that is involved in keeping us all healthy and well. Taking opioids from external sources in an acute situation such as needing pain relief is helpful; however, chronic use can interfere with the natural endo-opioids such as endorphins and enkephalins, which are needed for health.

Hallucinogens include marijuana, magic mushrooms, and LSD. Our bodies and brain also produce endocannabinoids such as anandamide that act on the cannabinoid receptors, which can be affected by hallucinogens coming from outside.

Organic solvents include things like glue and gasoline. These act on the brain more diffusely and can produce an alcohol-like intoxication, but they may also produce hallucinations as other brain structures get affected by higher dosages. Anaesthetic gases include diethyl ether (historically), enflurane (still used now), and nitrous oxide, and are inhalants that have medical uses but carry a potential for misuse and can become part of Addiction. Dissociative substances such as propofol and ketamine that are used intravenously produce a similar chemical effect through action on the n-methyl, d-aspartate (NMDA) receptor blockade. Hence, the initial euphoria resulting from disinhibition of neuronal circuits can turn into profound dissociation with perceptual distortions or hallucinations, with the final effect of death due to suppression of brain function essential to breathing.

All of these substances can be ingested by mouth and absorbed in the stomach; inhaled and absorbed through the lungs or the nose, if snorted; or injected intravenously (into the veins), intramuscularly (into the muscle), or intradermally (into the skin). They are all toxic to organs to varying degrees, with the organic solvents being irreversibly toxic to the brain. Some toxic effects on the liver, kidneys, and the hormonal system due to these substances can be reversible. All of these substances interfere with brain function such that there can be short- or long-term impairment in thinking, feeling, perception with the senses, and difficulties in motivation, memory, and acting responsibly in society, especially when low-risk using limits are exceeded. It is also important to appreciate that establishment of limits works only for people who do not have Addiction. People with Addiction will often exceed limits that are set by them or others, due to their inability to consistently abstain and impairment in behavioural control, which are characteristic of the underlying disease process. These can only be mitigated by proper treatment and ongoing continuing care in recovery, not by trying harder or setting stricter limits.

TOBACCO

The primary professional treatment intervention for Addiction involving tobacco or nicotine is not even classified as Addiction treatment by many providers and policy makers, as it has often focused squarely on the use of tobacco (nicotine) and on stopping that behaviour. Referred to as smoking cessation, this professional intervention has often used physicians or psychologists to assist people diagnosed with nicotine dependence to complete an analysis of their smoking behaviours. They look at the situations in which smoking is most likely to be engaged in and the conditioned cues that increase the likelihood of engaging in smoking. They then construct a system of rewards for success at reaching the goal of abstinence. Incremental reduction in quantity and frequency of tobacco use is more often accepted as a reasonable intermediate goal of behaviour change, yet many alcoholism counsellors would not embrace incremental reduction in the quantity and frequency of drinking as an intermediate treatment goal. These examples serve to demonstrate how even treatment providers get focused on what substances people are 'addicted to' rather than appreciating the broader manifestation of Addiction in a person's life. While abstinence from mind-altering substances is important for ongoing recovery, there are more implications for the disease and recovery than focusing on behaviour alone. For instance, without appreciating that someone has Addiction, it would be impossible to appreciate the spiritual, emotional, and cognitive warning signs that precede relapse. Thus, solely focusing on what people are 'addicted to' and their behaviour can actually make recovery, including abstinence, harder. Care providers have usually been trained in how to assist patients by motivational enhancement or brief office-based interventions. Some of the leading adoptees of these approaches have been family medicine physicians trained during residency programs by doctoral level psychologists on the use of such techniques.[1] Though Nicotine Anonymous exists, rarely are the group and family therapy techniques used in alcohol dependence treatment utilized in nicotine dependence treatment, despite it being the same disease. It used to be thought that nicotine dependence and tobacco addiction involved different circuitry than the full-blown disease of Addiction. However, clinical experience and research have demonstrated that children who have Addiction use tobacco as their initial drug to escape or alter moods. Some may stop at that if their disease is not too severe; however, most start to exhibit signs and symptoms of Addiction generally as they get older, especially with alcohol use problems or the D (Diminished recognition of problems in one's behaviours and interpersonal relationships) and E (dysfunctional Emotional response) characteristics of the disease of Addiction. This has profound implications for those trying to prevent the manifesta-tion of Addiction and its long-term complications. Preventing use of tobacco in our society is an essential intervention to decrease the devastation due to Addiction among individuals, families, communi-ties, and society.

In recent years, pharmacotherapy has been a central feature in the treatment of nicotine dependence. The use of nicotine replace-ment therapies has become so widespread that these have become over-the-counter drugs and they are used by many people in their own attempts at self-treatment without the assistance of a family physician, psychologist, or other professional. Arguably, nicotine replacement therapy treats withdrawal the same way opioid detoxi-fication or maintenance does, by allowing the person with Addiction to successfully maneuver his or her way through acute physiological withdrawal. This often opens the door for seeking other means of escape, reward, or relief. Newer pharmacotherapies such as the nico-tine receptor partial agonist agent, varenicline, address the Addictive disease itself, in addition to mitigating withdrawal symptoms. The presence of varenicline on the nicotine receptor decreases the craving for relief that is created when a receptor is sitting empty in wait for the anticipated nicotine through inhalation of tobacco smoke.

A clinical approach that views Addiction as a unitary condition recognizes that Addiction associated with nicotine and tobacco is the most deadly of all manifestations because of medical complica-tions such as emphysema and cancer.[2] Treatment providers need to make certain that all individuals have access to a full range of psy-chosocial and pharmacological therapies when people who are enter-ing recovery smoke. The group therapies utilized in the treatment of Addiction associated with alcohol, cocaine, and cannabis needs to be made available to persons with Addiction involving nicotine and tobacco. Family therapy interventions that are useful for treat-ment of Addiction can be utilized in cases of persons whose primary manifestation of Addiction appears to be their out-of-control use of tobacco products. Community-based mutual-help groups involving meeting with peers who share the goal of quitting smoking need to be utilized just as much as peer-support groups that have flourished for over seventy-five years for persons who share the goal of quitting drinking. It is important to emphasize that treatment of Addiction, of any form, needs to incorporate specific assessment and management interventions for the addictive use of tobacco products.

STIMULANTS AND CLUB DRUGS

Currently there is no FDA or Health Canada approved pharmacotherapy for the treatment of individuals with cocaine or other stimulant dependence; therefore, all professional interventions have been psychotherapeutic in nature. The same residential, partial hospitalization, intensive outpatient, and general outpatient approaches used for people diagnosed with alcohol, marijuana, or other drug dependence have been used with success for people whose primary source of reward or relief have been substances in the stimulant class of drugs. The significant threats to the public health posed by the cocaine epidemic of the 1980s and 1990s in North America led to intensive study, supported by federal research funding via the National Institute on Drug Abuse (NIDA),[3] into novel approaches that might offer enhanced results rather than treatment as usual. This research showed the strong influence of conditioned cues in the addictive process of individuals whose primary manifestation of Addiction was out-of-control use of cocaine or related pharmaceuticals and street drugs. This means that the environmental conditions associated with drug use were found to be a strong driver of ongoing drug use leading to inability to consistently abstain, in addition to the craving produced by alterations in neurochemicals in the brain. Relapse prevention therapies with a strong cognitive-behavioural component became quite popular, helping people identify the people, places, and things that seemed most powerful in triggering drug hunger and preoccupation and helping these people develop strategies to avoid such cues. Contingency management also has been found to be particularly helpful in many cases. This means that other rewards, such as monetary payment, are offered if there is demonstrated adherence to abstinence. NIDA-funded research has devoted quite a bit of attention to immunotherapies,[4] which block the ability of injected, smoked, or inhaled cocaine to reach and engage with reward circuitry in the brain. The immunotherapies focus largely on developing antibodies to the chemical such that the immune system of an individual who has received the vaccine would sequester the drug as soon as it enters the system. It cannot then produce the brain effects that the user would have been looking for. Pharmacotherapies for stimulant dependence to date have yielded disappointing results in attempting to manipulate the dopamine system with antidepressants, anti-Parkinsonian drugs, or amino acid precursors.

There is a notable rate of co-occurrence of stimulant and other substance dependence with sexual compulsivity, as well as with pathological gambling.[5] Though it has been hypothesized that people who prefer stimulants tend to seek enhanced excitement, stimulation, euphoria, and reward in contrast to people with alcohol or sedative-hypnotics as their primary substance who tend to seek relief of anxiety, depression, or existential angst, this is not a clear interaction. The reality is that people with Addiction seek reward and relief, sometimes focusing on lessening uncomfortable feelings or reinforcing positive ones at different points in the evolution of their illness. The contingency management and relapse-prevention approaches designed to help people with cocaine dependence are certainly useful for those with Addiction and need be considered for people with Addiction associated with alcohol, tobacco, gambling, spending, exercise, and other addictive behaviours, including other drugs.

ALCOHOL AND OTHER SEDATIVES

The broad availability of alcohol and its widespread social acceptance in many cultures is well established. Alcohol and other sedatives, such as benzodiazepines, z-drugs, such as zolpidem or zopiclone, and barbiturates, act as a depressant on the brain's function. They appear to be stimulants sometimes because they depress the inhibitory circuits in the brain. This means that the circuits that send messages to stop or slow down become impaired. This results in impulsivity or lack of restraint, together with the euphoria that is brought about through the opioid circuitry. Withdrawal symptoms from alcohol and other sedatives can vary from mild headache, nausea, and tremors to the more dangerous withdrawal seizures or delirium tremens for alcohol. If a person is experiencing the acute, more serious, and severe withdrawal symptoms, these need to be properly assessed and treated to prevent progression to seizures and delirium tremens.

Benzodiazepines remain the mainstay of acute withdrawal treatment, especially when there is a history of withdrawal seizures. Symptom-triggered withdrawal is the preferred method versus prescription of benzodiazepines on a fixed schedule for a variable number of days. This means that the medication is given to counteract the withdrawal symptoms acutely rather than substituting for any length of time with a fixed dosage that may be too much or too little. Both of these can increase the risk to relapse to active use of alcohol or sedatives. During treatment for alcohol dependence, when an individual is successful in abstaining from alcohol use through 'control' over this aspect of Addiction, the individual may actually be at increased risk for intensification in the pursuit of other unhealthy sources of reward or relief. For example, when alcohol, which had been increasing midbrain dopamine levels, is no longer available, there would be increasing symptoms of low dopamine, such as irritability and restlessness, which will drive the individual to seek other ways to activate the reward pathway in the brain. The conscious attempt to 'control' behaviours can lead to a 'hot condition' in which the brain and nervous system are focused on reward or relief, which has been shown to actually increase the likelihood of behavioural relapse. This means that abstaining from one substance, which one might see as success, is undermined by the appearance of other addictive behaviours because the brain just seeks the reward or relief through other means.

Case History: John. *John was very happy that he had been able to stop drinking for a month. He had also heard in AA that keeping candy or chocolate bars handy if a craving hit him was a good idea instead of turning to alcohol. He found himself looking for comfort in food on a regular basis. He was surprised to see that he had put on fifteen pounds in a month. John continued to find release and escape through eating and would turn to sweets whenever he was stressed or upset. Only when his counsellor challenged him on his Addiction involving food could he see this under the same umbrella as his use of alcohol.*

This is an example of how food can become the most effective reward or relief once alcohol abstinence is established.

Individuals who seek treatment for what they view as Addiction associated with alcohol and other sedatives use need to have tobacco use and other behaviours addressed by the professionals providing treatment. It is also essential to recognize that ongoing prescriptions for benzodiazepines or z-drugs, can be dangerous in preventing progress in recovery. Recurrent withdrawal symptoms due to changing blood levels of substance would exacerbate Addiction, and further increase the risk for post-acute withdrawal syndrome (PAWS), which is discussed further in Chapter 6.

OPIOIDS

Opioids are a group of drugs that act specifically on the opioid receptors that are found readily in various parts of the brain and body. Drugs such as morphine, codeine, and heroin that are derived from the opium poppy are opiates, whereas the synthetic drugs such as methadone and meperidine (Demerol) are not technically opiates. The term opioid is used to include opiates and the synthetics that act on the opioid receptor to produce an effect that appears to be desirable as a depressant but can also be energizing for some people. It certainly provides a level of relief or escape from pain, which is why opioids are commonly called painkillers. Interestingly, these drugs do not 'kill' pain; they just stop one from perceiving or caring about it. In acute injury situations that is a benefit while the body needs time to heal, but in chronic situations it can become a problem. These drugs are also called narcotics by some, which is erroneous because narcotics is a legal term referring to drugs on a controlled substance list that includes but is not limited to opioids. So, although opioids are on the narcotics list, not all narcotics are opioids.

Treatment of Addiction involving opioids in the past was primarily the treatment of inner-city intravenous heroin addicts, whereas now prescription opioids have become much more readily available, leading to more complications in terms of harmful use and Addiction. The multi-modal psychosocial interventions, often supplemented by ongoing community-based peer support found in Narcotics Anonymous groups, have been the mainstay for life-long abstinence and recovery. However, many clinics or agencies offering help to alcoholics do not embrace the patient with Addiction involving drugs, especially opioids. Relapse rates are often high for Addiction involving opioids because the withdrawal produces a high level of discomfort in terms of nausea, vomiting, gooseflesh, shivering, hot/cold flashes, diarrhea, and dysphoria, which pushes the affected individual to seek relief immediately rather than persevere through, even though opioid withdrawal is not life threatening. Natural opioids (endo-opioids) such as endorphins and enkephalins produced by the body to maintain health and wellbeing also may become deficient with chronic use of opioids. The presence of these external opioids in the system interferes with the natural production such that the system takes time to recover over months rather than days. This creates a level of dysphoria even in the absence of other symptoms that takes the affected individual back to taking opioids. Long-term, meaning twelve months or more, residential treatment services were developed in the form of therapeutic communities to address this problem. Therapeutic communities are treatment campuses where low intensity treatment is provided in an environment that is relatively stress-free and keeps the people with Addiction engaged in routine chores in community living, thus helping them deal with their feelings and past issues as they develop recovery skills in a low-intensity therapeutic setting. This time also allows the natural endorphin/enkephalin system to recalibrate.

As the resources required for long-term residential therapy are not always available and people's willingness or ability to live long-term in such a community is not always present, maintenance pharmacotherapy has been a more accepted approach in persons with Addiction involving opioids. Through extensive research, it has also been found that agonist (such as methadone) and partial agonist (such as buprenorphine) therapy has been more successful in preventing relapse. Agonist means that the medication acts on the same receptor as the drug being used by person with Addiction in the same manner to provide the same result, which prevents withdrawal symptoms and thus the pursuit of opioids on the street. A partial agonist means that the effect is less than a full agonist and may carry a ceiling dose. This is the case with buprenorphine. The danger is that many patients and providers mistakenly believe that opioid maintenance is correcting the so-called opioid deficiency in opioid dependence and often the broader aspects of addiction-related problems are overlooked. Opioid dependence is sometimes treated with an antagonist such as naloxone in a rapid opioid detox setting. An antagonist means the substance acts on the same receptor as the agonist but produces a receptor blocking effect, which triggers withdrawal. The rationale for using naloxone is to flush the opioids out, but the procedure alone is not Addiction treatment. Naltrexone, which is a long acting opioid antagonist, may be given in an oral, depot injection or pellet implant form to continue the blockade of opioid receptors to prevent craving. Relapse rates remain high through this route of care, unless broader aspects of Addiction are addressed in a treatment program.

The two most common maintenance therapies for treatment of opioid Addiction are methadone, which is a long-acting full agonist, and buprenorphine, which is a long-acting partial agonist. Buprenorphine maintenance in North America is usually done with a sublingual (under the tongue) formulation such as Suboxone, where naloxone is added to the buprenorphine. Naloxone is an opioid antagonist, which can bring about withdrawal by displacing agonist medication from the opioid receptors. However, it is only active when given intravenously. Hence, in the sublingual formulation the naloxone is largely inert. The addition of naloxone discourages intravenous use as the antagonist effect comes into play if one injects Suboxone rather than taking it sublingually as prescribed. There is no overdose risk with buprenorphine because of it being a partial agonist, but there is significant risk of overdose if it is used with alcohol or other sedatives. The long-acting nature of methadone presents an overdose risk. Patients needing naloxone to reverse an opioid overdose involving methadone need to be given repeated injections of naloxone, as it is short acting, or they may need to be on a naloxone intravenous drip in the hospital until the methadone levels have become non-threatening. Someone presenting with a methadone overdose can die at home if they are released after the overdose is reversed, only by a single injection of naloxone in the Emergency Room.

The long-term residential approaches or agonist maintenance treatment found necessary for many persons with Addiction involving opioids may be necessary for some persons with other aspects of Addiction, where recurrent relapses occur in the context of chronic, entrenched problems. These approaches are not limited to those who use opioids as part of their Addiction, because agonist maintenance treatment is common for Addiction involving tobacco with nicotine replacement therapy. A therapeutic community may be also the preferred treatment for people with severe alcohol dependence or cocaine dependence who experience recurrent relapses in the context of having severe disease biologically or unstable psycho-social-spiritual circumstances that interfere with their engagement in meaningful recovery when living in general society.

MARIJUANA AND OTHER HALLUCINOGENS

Cannabis use is common in our society today, with or without the use of other hallucinogens such as magic mushrooms or LSD. Marijuana use is often downplayed by calling it a 'soft drug' when, in fact, chronic marijuana use leads to accumulation of the substance in the body and brain so that an individual will test positive for the substance over long periods, which may stretch to as long as a few months. The effects of cannabis on memory circuits acutely and chronically are sometimes difficult to appreciate fully and the effects on and research related to interference with the endo-cannabinoid circuitry is ongoing.[6] Cannabis withdrawal is being recognized now and may persist in individuals for long periods in the form of irritability, poor concentration, and memory problems. Marijuana use likely interferes with the production and balance of endo-cannabinoids that are essential for the body's natural balance in maintaining health and well-being.

Abstinence from marijuana use needs to be an essential component even of agonist maintained treatment options such as opioid agonist therapy or nicotine maintenance therapy. Healthy recovery is an elusive goal in the presence of the reward circuitry being stimulated on an ongoing basis by marijuana. In other words, Addiction treatment is less likely to be effective if people are still smoking marijuana or engaging in any other substance use during the process. Although some advocate marijuana maintenance as a 'lesser of other evils', it is not a recognized or effective form of treatment for Addiction.

INHALANTS

Inhalants[7] are volatile substances such as gasoline, paint thinner, glue, and aerosol propellant gases. They can be inhaled as vapors through plastic bags held over the mouth or by breathing from an open container. This is called huffing, sniffing, or bagging. Nitrous oxide gases from whipped cream aerosol cans, aerosol hairspray, or non-stick frying spray can be sprayed into other containers or on rags to sniff the vapors. The inhalants have a quick effect on the brain because of rapid absorption through extensive capillary surface of the lungs. The intensity of effects is similar to that achieved by intravenous injection.

Inhalant intoxication can vary widely depending on the dose and what type of solvent or gas is inhaled, from being somewhat impaired or intoxicated to more severe dissociation, where hallucinations, distortion in perceptions of time and space, and emotional disturbances can occur. Headache, nausea, and vomiting, slurred speech, loss of coordination or motor control, and wheezing as an acute effect can occur as well. Prolonged use often produces a characteristic glue sniffer's rash around the nose and mouth. Paint or solvent residues can sometimes emerge in sweat after the person has used, which can be recognized by others. Inhalants can result in acute problems with disruptions in heart rhythm or breathing that can be fatal. They can also cause serious harm to the brain, kidneys, and liver over the long term among regular users who have Addiction and are unable or unwilling to abstain.

Inhalants are a common problem among marginalized adolescent populations around the world who are isolated, impoverished, and without hope or means to deal with their unfortunate circumstances. In Canada, the homeless and isolated communities among First Nations people most widely face these challenges among their children. In the 1990s, the northern native community of Davis Inlet in Canada became well known for the number of children affected by huffing. Treatment interventions remain difficult even today because

the systemic change that is required for ongoing recovery is not supported by the current government or community infrastructures.

GAMBLING

In our society, gambling takes many forms, including casual betting,
lottery tickets, video lottery terminals (VLTs), casinos and 'get rich
quick' investments. Internet gambling is readily accessible as well. It
is essential that questions related to gambling are asked during an
assessment for Addiction, regardless of the presenting substance(s)
or behaviour(s) that may have brought the individual forward in
seeking help. Gambling leads to grave financial consequences beyond
the money spent on specific drugs or behaviours as large amounts of
money can be lost very quickly. Lines of credit related to the matri-
monial home or cashing in retirement savings for cash to gamble and
subsequent losses are devastating to families. Not addressing this in
those treated for Addiction involving substances is a big contributor to suicide in individuals who carry a tremendous shame burden
even when they may be maintaining abstinence from the use of
psychoactive substances. It is essential to appreciate the role of the
chase,[8] which is obvious and rewarding in the case of gambling, as
being reinforcement for Addiction. The pursuit of reward, more so
than the actual acquisition, is what is rewarding. Therefore, a person
may be vulnerable even if they have not acted out because they
were in pursuit of their next hit, even though they never acquired
it. For example, someone who spent hours plotting how they would
get to the local strip mall to buy lottery tickets but was unable to
find money to purchase the tickets. The rewarding effect of pursuit
applies to all aspects of Addiction and is a big driver of behaviour.
Those without a full understanding of Addiction may miss this and
congratulate the person for 'stopping the behaviour,' although they
received just as strong of a dopamine hit as if they had acted out.

Treatment and recovery need to address the bottom-line behaviours that would characterize abstinence on an individual basis.

Bottom-line behaviours refer to those that are compulsive, feed the disease, and that need to be abstained from for the individual to get better. For example, although someone may present as wanting to get well from Addiction involving gambling, they will also need to look at all other aspects of their life. Their behavioural recovery would involve setting bottom-line behaviours related to gambling and spending. For example, not going to casinos, purchasing lottery tickets, or doing online poker, as well as having a budget each month for expenses and fun purchases. Additionally, quitting alcohol and smoking, reducing consumption of sugar and processed foods, and limiting sexual activity to that within the context of a relationship rather than including frequent masturbation and casual sexual encounters, would need to be explored.

EATING DISORDERS

A myriad of food-related issues can arise during adolescence and young adulthood that can range from anorexia, binging, purging, and persistent overeating as an escape or reward-seeking response to emotional stressors, resulting in obesity over a short or long period.

Obesity is not always the result of Addiction. There are other metabolic pathways that can be involved with obesity that do not involve the midbrain reward circuit. Historically, however, Addiction has been greatly under-diagnosed in obesity treatment. The large increase in literature relating to the onset of opioid or alcohol dependence or 'new onset Addiction' in women post-bariatric surgery is an important example of this. Rather than having been seen as patients with Addiction, some patients were seen as having pathologies of gastric signaling systems. Gastric manipulation was shown to affect those signaling systems, and various forms of gastric procedures were logically used as interventions.[9] If the patients had only been suffering from the proposed gastric signaling pathologies, the story would have ended there. However, not surprisingly, several researchers have shown a large increase in incidence of Addiction following such procedures. If the patients had Addiction and were using food as a source of reward, the phenomenon would not have been seen as the new onset of Addiction, but rather as the expected switch to a new drug when the illness is not treated but the drug of food is made unavailable.

Some have suggested other mechanisms to explain this new onset of Addiction following gastric shortening while trying to keep an Addiction-free paradigm of obesity. One such explanation is that these people have been newly exposed to opioids because of the surgical procedure and had increased risk because of that exposure. Another is that gastric shortening decreased the length of the path to highest alcohol absorption and therefore increased the speed of absorption and reward from alcohol. These explanations seem to be adding to the complexity of the Gordian knot rather than sharpening Occam's razor. In other words, these explanations create unnecessary confusion and complexity rather than allowing the most straightforward answer to be understood. When unexpected results occur from a procedure for poorly understood pathology, the most likely cause is a fault in the initial hypothesis. Addiction involving food, in the context of an eating disorder, is the pathology that cannot be corrected surgically. As interference occurs with food absorption post-surgically, it is not surprising that opioids would become the most effective reward in some, whereas others may turn to alcohol. Clinically, we have seen this problem with patients losing weight after bariatric surgery, only to get into difficulties with Addiction involving alcohol or opioids.

Another hint that obesity and compulsive overeating can be a manifestation of Addiction is the long history of the effectiveness of stimulants or dopamine-raising medications as weight loss medications. There is also the example of the common weight gain that happens after stopping tobacco use. This is not related to metabolic changes so much as changes in eating patterns. One way or the other, the low-dopamine brain will seek out sources of dopamine in the environment.

Eating disorders also highlight the other major aspect of Addiction that involves 'all or nothing' thinking and behaviours that are connected with anorexia or binging, together with purging with vomiting, laxatives, or exercise at times to counteract the effects of binging. Hence, it is essential to talk to people with Addiction about food issues rather than making assumptions that there is no problem if the individual is not overweight or denies overeating. The fellowship of Anorexics and Bulimics Anonymous[10] addresses the needs of people with Addiction involving food that do not relate to overeating behaviour, which is addressed Overeaters Anonymous groups.

SEXUAL DISORDERS

Sexual behaviours are stigmatized in Western society even when they are within normal ranges; therefore, abnormal sexual behaviours have been difficult to discuss, assess, and treat. A variety of sexual behaviours exist that are not the median or mode in terms of frequency of the activity, but may be part of the repertoire of a person. As more has been understood about people who engage in sexual activity that has an out-of-control quality, it has been necessary to differentiate between the out-of-control and the unusual. People whose behaviour is out-of-control follow the Addiction pattern, such that there is a great deal of time, effort, and resources put into obtaining and participating in the behaviours; there are significant consequences for the behaviours; and there is an inability to stop the behaviours without help in spite of a desire to do so. The behavioural treatment is also similar to treatment for Addiction involving substances, although it has usually been provided in specialized programs that may or may not insist on abstinence from the use of psychoactive substances.

Where therapists and doctors need help with treatment provision has to do with how our society struggles to talk about sexual behaviour more so than learning about specific interventions unique to Addiction involving sex. Abstinence is usually not the long-term goal in the treatment of Addiction involving sex, love, and relationships. However, an initial three-month period of complete abstinence is often necessary to establish a foundation of recovery. In early recovery, it is difficult for the affected individual to distinguish whether the desire for sex is in the context of a healthy relationship or it is connected to escape or avoidance of feelings. Goals, in recovery, are set around sexual behaviours that can be done without shame or compromise of values. Slips into compulsive behaviour are to be anticipated and are used to re-draw boundaries and re-establish goals. This work is done in residential, partial hospitalization, intensive outpatient, or traditional outpatient settings. Participation in sex-specific 12-step groups[11] is also useful. This participation helps to drastically reduce shame and opens up dialogue about behaviours that would otherwise remain a secret. Involvement of sexual partners in therapy is also quite important so that both people can work together to develop a sexual relationship that is supportive of recovery.

Additional treatment options may include the judicious use of a well-trained and experienced therapist who utilizes eye movement desensitization and reprocessing (EMDR) or a hypnotherapist to uncover secrets not yet revealed in therapy, such as trauma, abuse, or other experiences that may affect health and behaviour. Medications useful for Addiction involving sex include those that lower libido. Anti-depressants, such as selective serotonin reuptake inhibitors (SSRIs), are most commonly used but there is not yet a body of literature supporting this. Anti-craving medications, particularly naltrexone, have been shown to be useful in clinical experience. Long-term, people define their own abstinence consistent with their vulnerabilities, which usually consists of no masturbation, pornography, or sexual acting out even in fantasy, and having sex only in the context of a monogamous relationship, as triggers can easily take people back to old established routines connected with Addiction if these boundaries are not drawn.

RELATIONSHIPS

The ASAM definition of Addiction has identified "Diminished recognition of significant problems in one's behaviours and interpersonal relationships" as the D in the ABCDE characteristics of the disease. It is essential to assess the relationship dysfunction in every individual from the perspectives of relationship with self, others, and a higher power that cover the biological, psychological, social, and spiritual dimensions. The relationship with oneself and critical examination of behaviours are essential aspects of recovery and necessary in developing healthy relationships with others. Cultivation of awareness of one's relationship with a higher power provides a broader, universal, existential perspective to the interaction with others as well.

As much as the diagnosis of borderline personality disorder[12] is used for individuals chronically affected by persistent problems in relationships, the recovery context is helpful in addressing those behaviours and encouraging more realistic and balanced relationships. Transference and counter-transference issues also contribute to relationship problems, especially in interaction with treatment providers. For instance, individuals who were raised by a neglectful and emotionally distant father may be challenged in working with a male treatment provider and find themselves reacting to that provider as they would have their father. Likewise, treatment providers who have been around individuals who are reactive, hostile, and conflict-oriented might find it difficult to work with patients exhibiting strong relationship issues.

The relationship with a significant other or spouse is an important social relationship to address in recovery. Assertiveness and boundary issues need to be explored during treatment on an ongoing basis to ensure that there is a healthy balance between meeting one's own needs and honoring the needs of others in a mutually supportive, interdependent manner, rather than demanding or controlling behaviours filled with manipulation, expectations, and resentments related to the unmet expectations that characterize dysfunction. Avoidance of fantasy and projection is necessary to ensure that social interactions and relationships are grounded in the reality of 'what is' as opposed to 'what should/could be.' Projection means putting one's own feelings onto another. One example is saying, 'Why are you so resentful?' to your spouse when you are the one who is carrying resentments.

We are social creatures and relationships are an integral part of the human experience. People all have dependency needs and this can be achieved in healthy relationships that foster growth and self-esteem. They allow people to be accepted for who they are and there is reciprocity between the individuals. Reciprocal relationships require a spirit of cooperation, as well as an understanding of and ability to embrace interdependence. Interdependence in a healthy relationship requires that both people accept personal responsibility. One person cannot take all the blame while the other person gives it all. Acceptance of responsibility for the creation of a reciprocal relationship takes a high degree of emotional maturity, personal awareness, and time to develop. Interdependence is essential to any healthy relationship and can be defined as staying true to one self, having boundaries that are firm yet flexible, and knowing when and how to give help or to say no. It is about caring and giving to others but doing so with consciousness and compassion, not martyrdom, and with enough self-awareness of when to pull back before it negatively affects your own health and wellbeing.

The definition of codependence[13] has been varied in the literature and it remains ambiguous. Originally, codependence was used to describe persons living with someone who is chemically dependent. In AA circles, codependence has often been equated with the partner of the alcoholic and the person attending Al-Anon meetings. When the term codependent was originally coined, it was defined in the context of Al-Anon as someone whose life had become unmanageable as a result of living in a relationship with an alcoholic.

When assessing an individual's alcohol intake, it can be helpful to visualize the continuum of use pictured below (Figure 3). On the one end of the continuum, there is no use, followed by low risk use, abuse, and then crossing the 'pickle line' over to Addiction or dependence.

No Use...Low Risk Use...Substance Abuse...|...Addiction/Dependence

The Pickle Line
A cucumber can become a pickle but a pickle can't
go back to become a cucumber

FIGURE 3 THE PICKLE LINE

This continuum is also helpful when discussing relationships (Figure 4). It shows healthy, interdependent relationships on one end, then codependence and crossing the pickle line to relationship Addiction. Codependence is seen in a similar light to alcohol abuse because both occur when the individual demonstrates unhealthy behaviours that are detrimental to their overall health and wellbeing. As humans, we are all vulnerable to codependent relationships and, in some situations, we may unconsciously display unhealthy patterns of reacting and coping, which needs to be explored further in treatment and differentiated from Addiction involving relationships.

Healthy interdependent......Codependent...|...Addiction involving
relationships

The Pickle Line
A cucumber can become a pickle but a pickle can't
go back to become a cucumber

FIGURE 4 THE RELATIONSHIP CONTINUUM

In Addiction involving relationships, compulsive behaviours are evident in connection with people such as an intimate partner, parent, child, or friends. The person with Addiction demonstrates behaviour similar to being intoxicated, which can be referred to as relationship intoxication. Relationship intoxication occurs when an individual feels good and gets a high when they get some of their needs met through a relationship but it is never enough and there is a continued desire for more. The person with Addiction may become needy and manipulative to get their needs met but they continue to feel unsatisfied.

With Addiction involving relationships, it is common for people with Addiction to feel withdrawal when the relationship has ended or the partner is absent for a while. In withdrawal, there may be heightened anxiety, depression, sadness, fear, shame, or irritability. For example, if their partner goes away for a business trip, the person with Addiction will text and call multiple times per day to check-in. When they are not phoning or sending messages, the person with Addiction worries and script writes about what their partner is doing, where they are, what they are thinking, and how they are feeling. People with Addiction involving relationships can experience high levels of paranoia, worried that any absence or delay in response means their partner has left, stopped loving them, or that they are cheating. The fantasy aspect of relationship is akin to the importance of the chase concept discussed earlier, with the chase being more reinforcing than the acquisition. As you can see, there are many parallels between the unmanageability, obsession, and compulsion in Addiction involving substances and Addiction involving relationships. This is evidence for it being the same disease as Addiction involving substances. The 'drug of choice' or most effective reward is relationships, where people affected will even rationalize to the point of believing that an abusive relationship is better than none.

With Addiction involving relationships, the affected individual may try to control the other person in order to feel okay and get their needs met. Rather than respect the other person's separateness and individuality, they cannot tolerate disagreement and blame the other for causing their problems without taking responsibility for themselves. For example, 'It is your fault I feel paranoid because you did not pick up the phone when I called.' The relationship becomes dysfunctional and out of balance. There are frequent struggles for power and control in Addiction involving relationships. Sometimes what they dislike in their partner is the very thing they cannot accept in themselves. For instance, while you may be ventilating about your spouse not being able to communicate their feelings adequately, you have a difficult time assertively expressing your own. Despite their pain, the person with Addiction can feel trapped in the relationship because they fear that they cannot function on their own. The person with Addiction's insecurity also makes intimacy threatening, since being honest with their partner risks rejection and dissolution of the fragile self.

Knowledge of recovery and what is needed for change does not necessarily alter behaviours. Action is the essential component of recovery and this can occur with or without knowledge. Knowledge grows with action, which then leads to more awareness and further action. For example, someone may not understand why their health care provider is recommending they abstain from masturbation for a minimum of three months and may not be aware what benefit this will have for them. Rather than waiting until they understand and are aware, it is important to take action and, in so doing, can come to a greater knowledge of what benefit and purpose this serves. In this instance, one learns from abstaining that they were using masturbation to mood-alter; they might develop greater awareness of the unmanageability of masturbation in their life; or may realize the distancing effect it had in the relationship. Whatever the case may be, these realizations would not have been possible without action.

'Can't they see how much they are hurting themselves and everyone around them?' 'Why don't they just stop, what is wrong with them?' All too often, this is the approach of family, friends, health care professionals, and even patients with the disease of Addiction. Rather, considering Addiction as a brain disease and a condition involving impairment in behavioural control means that what is wrong with the person is not what they are doing, or what they could do, but how their brain responds to exposure to substances or activities that activate their reward, motivation, memory, and related circuitry.

Relationships, particularly in the context of Addiction, are complex and difficult to understand in terms of what is healthy or not. In relationships, it is important to understand the roles that are taken on, which is further discussed in the chapter for family members. There are also tools, like the Karpman Triangle, that help us make sense out of our behaviour and get a clearer understanding of what is healthy for us in relationships.

THE KARPMAN DRAMA TRIANGLE

The Karpman Drama Triangle is a psychological concept that comes out of transactional analysis (TA) theory, first described by Dr. Stephen B. Karpman in 1968. [14] It describes the roles that individuals may take in a situation (Figure 5). Once an individual takes on one of the roles, the other person usually follows suit by taking on another role in the triangle. From there, they may switch to different roles as the interaction continues. Proponents of TA refer to the triangle as a mind game that people play when interacting with other.

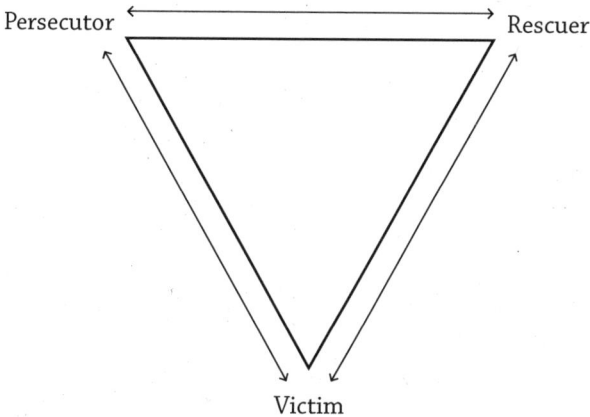

FIGURE 5 THE KARPMAN DRAMA TRIANGLE

The victim is the individual who feels attacked or persecuted by others. They will often ventilate or complain about the situations and circumstances currently being faced, while taking on a passive role. Things are happening to the victim that they believe they cannot influence. The persecutor pressures, coerces, or threatens the victim in some way. The persecutor takes on an aggressive stance and can be confrontational and bullying.

Often a victim will become a persecutor, if given time and enough emotional ammunition, as they reach their boiling point. This starts up a strange dance in which both the persecutor and the victim see the other as the problem and neither is able or willing to look at their own role in perpetuating the unhealthy dynamic in the relationship.

The rescuer, who may come in seemingly to help or save the victim, is actually motivated by their own ego rather than a pure desire to provide support. There may be a dishonest or mixed motive behind the offer of help with some secondary gain, whether that is monetary, sexual, or otherwise. This may not be the conscious intent of the rescuer, but it operates at a subconscious or unconscious level. In other words, it is not unconditional support because there are strings attached in the form of benefits for the rescuer. Thus, the rescuer becomes a persecutor or perpetrator, thus further reinforcing the role for the victim. In dysfunctional relationships and friendships, the drama continues with everybody feeling victimized while trying to rescue others and becoming perpetrators of more emotional abuse towards each other. Any of these roles have the ability to generate shame and perpetuate a life of unhealthiness and dysfunction within oneself and in relationships.

It is essential to realize that all three roles can be played by the same individual, depending on circumstances and relationships, which often gets labeled as 'we are all human' when it actually is the dance of dysfunction where everyone stays ill rather than looking at the problem realistically and seeking definitive solutions. Self-awareness and accepting feedback from others are essential to recognize where one may be on the triangle in any given relationship that has become dysfunctional.

Anytime one finds themselves on this triangle, it is important to step back and ask, 1) What is the motivation for my behaviour? 2) How am I feeling? and 3) What is the real issue here? Doing so will help move you into the healthy relationship pattern of helper, protector, and survivor (Figure 6).

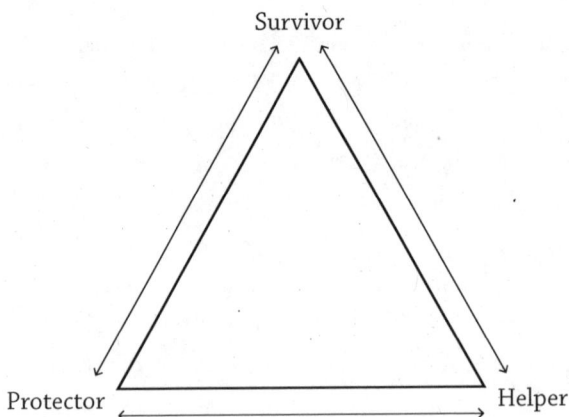

FIGURE 6 RECOVERY ROLES

The victim can be assisted in moving towards the survivor through professional treatment and support from peers, friends, and family. Finding their voice through assertiveness, affirmations, and raising self-esteem are empowering for the victim. The rescuer can become a true helper by connecting with their own needs and establishing healthy boundaries that are congruent with this. For example, this may mean not providing financial support for a struggling loved one but offering to take them to a 12-step meeting instead. The persecutor can become a protector or supporter such that there is unconditional support with honest communication, accountability, and responsibility.

ENVIRONMENT, EXPOSURE, AND STRESS

In 12-step circles, it is anecdotally discussed that there are three major ways to relapse. These have long been referred to as people, places, and things. More recently, ASAM has incorporated these concepts into the definition of Addiction, as brain research has established the circuitry associated with these pathways. In the ASAM definition they are known as environment, exposure and stress. If one, two, or all three of these factors are present in the person's life at any time, their vulnerability for addictive thinking and spiritual, emotional, cognitive, social, and behavioural relapse increases. With further scientific research, more is now known about how these make people vulnerable.

Environment. The environment pathway refers to places that remind people of using and active Addiction. Examples of risky places that focus the brain back on disease rather than reinforcing recovery include places where using happened in the past, such as bars. For solitary drinkers, the home alone scenario would be a trigger, as well as special events such as weddings or funerals. Even work, which can serve as a distraction and keep you busy may increase vulnerability after work or be an environment associated with drinking at lunch or alone in the office at the end of the day.

Studies have shown that it takes only milliseconds of exposure to these cues to activate the brain's pleasure/reward centre. This means that vulnerability increases at the level of the brain faster than is known to conscious awareness. This is also the reason that testing oneself by purposefully being in risky environments and hoping for the best can be extremely risky and result in the worst outcome, which is relapse, or the second worst outcome, which is that there is no immediate relapse but the brain is cued to wanting escape, reward, or relief. The person in recovery thinks they are safe, but if the disease of Addiction has been activated in the brain, acting out may follow some hours or days later. Relapse or relapse warning signs may persist for days, weeks, or months after exposure to environments, substances, problem behaviour, or stress. The brain reacts quickly to environments and triggers escape, relief, or reward cues, which can be frustrating and confusing to the person in recovery, as shown by Vanessa's story.

Case History: Vanessa. 'I feel like crawling out of my skin when I am home alone,' says Vanessa, who has been in recovery for six months. 'Especially in my living room. Whenever I go sit down to watch TV in my favourite chair, I feel so uncomfortable. I even start to sweat a little. What is wrong with me? I think I'm going crazy. Who can't sit and watch TV in their living room without wanting to drink?'

'Where would you typically drink when you were in active Addiction, Vanessa?' asks the therapist.

Vanessa thinks for a moment and shakes her head in disbelief. 'Right in that chair. My ritual was that I would come home from work and my family would still be out, so I would pour myself a drink in this big, plastic flowery cup that my daughter has and drink and watch TV until they came home. That's crazy, though. Are you saying that my body wants a drink just because I'm sitting in that chair?'

Vanessa has already answered her own question. She is now aware that simply being in the environment where she once used can cause the body to crave using and respond as though she is—in this case, by sweating. Other physical signs may include heart racing, hands shaking, lips trembling, and shortness of breath. This is the body reacting to that environment at a base physiological level. Vanessa in recovery is not craving or even thinking consciously about alcohol, but her brain has been conditioned that 'when I sit in this chair, I drink.' Because this happens so fast, it is important to be mindful of old using environments and to minimize exposure as much as possible. If this is not possible, having strong recovery support with you or available, as well as an exit strategy if things take a turn to the risky.

Exposure. Theoretically, exposure can involve people, places, and things that trigger the brain to be reminded of the active disease state and begin sending the message that it wants that again. Exposure means contact with a risky person, environment, substance, object, emotion, or behaviour with any of the five senses.

Smell and Taste. Smell and taste have long been known to be the senses most strongly associated with memory. This is why certain perfumes, foods, or odours have the ability to instantly bring us back to a past time or situation, perhaps without our even being aware of this. The person in recovery who takes a whiff of vintage wine because they like the smell is under the spell of their disease, which is enticing them to get closer to their vulnerability and telling them it is okay to just have a whiff. People have acknowledged smelling liquor sitting in a locked cabinet in the living room, though they had previously denied that alcohol in the home was a trigger. For this reason, it is important to have an alcohol-free home. Flavoured foods or beverages that mimic the taste of alcohol in its various forms such as rum or whiskey flavoured desserts can also act as triggers for renewed craving, even if no alcohol is actually there.

Handling substances, even without the intention of consuming them, is playing a dangerous game with the disease of Addiction. Exposure through other senses (sight, smell, sound) become cued, which may lead to the worst or second-worst outcome.

People in recovery can easily become caught in the trap of think-ing, 'I can handle just one.' This is a false message that is sent from the Addiction part of the brain. Once someone has crossed the pickle line into dependence, the ability to control drinking is false evidence appearing real. A person may think they are able to drink moder-ately, and perhaps they can for a period of time, but the disease is progressive and ever-present and, eventually, things will spiral out of control. People may also convince themselves that small tastes or sips are harmless, but it is important to consider that there is still risk and harm involved; it just may be that direct, observable conse-quences do not immediately occur.

Sight. A substance of choice, a person that was involved in using, a place that reminds one of using, or advertisements for gambling, alcohol, slimness, etc.—the list of visual vulnerabilities goes on and can include a number of different people, places, or things. Visual cues are registered quickly by the brain and, much like other sensory inputs, register faster than the conscious brain can pick up. While a person may feel they have escaped safely after being visually exposed to stimuli associated with their Addiction, there was likely mental activation that will increase vulnerability for days, weeks, or months after exposure.

Hearing and Touch. Advertising on the radio is great at generat-ing imagery that engages the brain from a memory perspective, thus driving thinking, feeling, and behaviour. A radio ad developed many years ago, supposedly for responsible drinking, had sounds related to a family picnic and a voiceover saying, 'Everyone has their reasons for drinking, have you thought about yours? Please drink responsi-bly.' For someone with Addiction, this would trigger a euphoric recall of good times that could easily lead to rationalization and relapse. The advertising consultants know that the way to motivate someone to engage in behaviours is to remind them of something associ-ated with pleasure. An advertisement for responsible drinking may actually promote drinking and becomes dangerous for those with Addiction. Similarly, touching a cold bottle or glass of beer has been known to trigger cravings in individuals that had been successfully abstinent for years because of the instant flood of memories it can bring back.

Pat's experience is a great example of the impact that environment and exposure can have on an individual. He had a strong recovery foundation of multiple 12-step meetings per week, working with a sponsor, doing regular group and individual therapy, and being aware of Addiction and addictive thinking. Thanks to that regime, the worst outcome did not happen, which would have been drinking. However, Pat experienced the second worst outcome: increased disease activity and discomfort that took a few weeks to calm down.

Case History: Pat. *'I went to a wedding for the first time without my wife last week,' Pat, sober from alcohol for three years, shares in a psychotherapy session. 'I wanted to try it and see what would happen, as she has been my source of support for these last few years of recovery. I wanted to do it on my own.'*

'And what happened?' asks the therapist.

Pat shakes his head and laughs. 'Nothing. Not at the time, anyway. Well, not nothing, it was hard. Liquor was flowing all around me and then the table of shots came out. I knew at that point in the evening I had to leave, so I went back to my room. I made it. I got through without drinking even though my wife was not there.'

'How did you feel when you came back from the wedding?'

Pat laughs again. 'Horrible! I was cranky, snapping at my wife for no reason, wanting to disconnect from the family again just like I had when I was drinking. But that was the thing: I hadn't touched a drop of alcohol. You know how I have been trying to cut down on eating candy and sweets? Yeah, that didn't go so well this week either. My brain is going haywire after that trip.'

This example shows how impactful exposure to substance can be, even if the substance itself is not consumed. An additional vulnerability in the disease of Addiction is to the feelings associated with stress.

Stress. When people hear the word stress, they often associate it as being bad. This label has been misattributed to stress, conveying the message that if you feel any discomfort you would identify it as stress and then you need to make it go away because this is bad. Stress can be destructive and uncomfortable, particularly if it is intense or persists for a long period. Most times, however, stress benefits us and helps us function. Stress is a message from our body and is a source of information; therefore, it is important to listen and deal with it in a healthy way, not ignore, control, manage, or avoid it.

Stress is an organism's total response to environmental demands or pressures or, more simply, it is how people respond to life. The relationship between performance and stress has been graphed in the Yerkes-Dobson 'inverted U' (Figure 7).

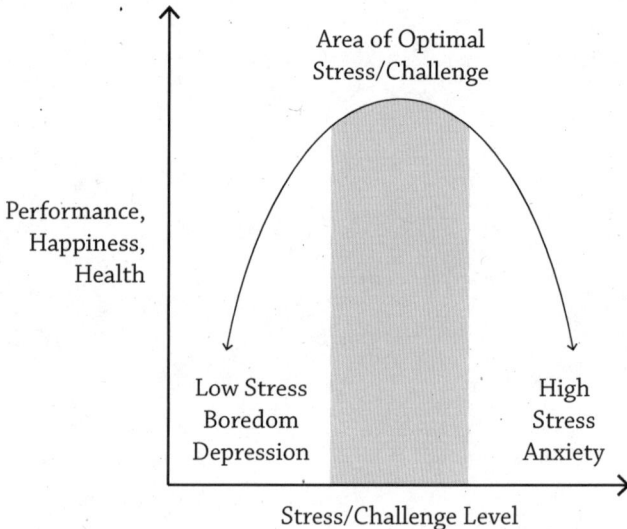

FIGURE 7 THE PERFORMANCE-STRESS INVERTED 'U'

Stress is a natural response to our environment and helps motivate us and keep us functioning. Without some degree of stress, people would be listless and aimless in life. Too much stress, on the other hand, will have physical and psychological implications. People feel uncomfortable, experience difficulty concentrating and with decision-making, have impairment in memory, and often a desire to seek relief from these experiences and the situations causing them.

Stress can be acute or chronic. Acute stressors are sudden in onset, usually have a defined beginning and end, and do not last long. Examples of acute stressors include a broken limb, a traffic jam, or a work project. A chronic stressor is one that continues for a long period (e.g., chronic illness, pain, divorce). Our natural response to stress (real or perceived) is to *fight, flight,* or *freeze.*

The fight response includes increased conflict, arguments, and even verbal or physical aggression. Often in fight mode, people want to fix or control the stressful situation, which is not always possible or in one's best interests. For example, if Ross is stressed because his thirty-year-old daughter, Rosa, is unhappy in her marriage, confronting Rosa's husband does not change their marital relationship, and increases tension between Rosa and Ross, which increases his overall stress level.

The flight response is avoiding or minimizing the problem(s). Again, this response can increase stress because stressors, such as bills or conflicts, can only be avoided for so long. Both of the options of fight or flight are enticing for the addicted mind because they produce immediate relief or escape. However, they can increase stress if things are not dealt with and the situation builds over time.

The third and less commonly talked about response to stress is to freeze. Think of a deer in the headlights that is in such shock looking at an oncoming vehicle that their mind cannot decide what to do. They may be stuck trying to decide, 'Do I run, or do I stay put?' The same thing can happen with people, which is called analysis paralysis. People become so caught up in analyzing the situation and trying to determine the right course of action that they become frozen and end up doing nothing. Again, this often only serves to increase stress because the situation still exists and is not being addressed.

The most amazing thing is that the situations that cause stress are not always inherently stressful. Our perception of events plays a major role in the experience of stress. For example, does a traffic jam have to be stressful? No. It is the labelling and attached meaning that makes it so. It is important to remember that stress will eventually go away and does not last forever; rather, it is a function of life that ebbs and flows. The more one focuses on stress as a negative experience, the longer it will last and the more detrimental it will be. If one can work on accepting the messages stress is communicating, then balance can be restored.

With healthy coping skills, the impact of stress on self can be lessened. It is like a current—it can pull you in the more you fight or carry you along if you accept it as a natural part of life. With a healthy lifestyle that has a bio-psycho-social-spiritual focus, stress can be lessened. Having other ways of coping helps the brain by developing alternate pathways that reinforce recovery, thus mitigating the impact of relapse forces on the brain.

ADDICTION IS ADDICTION

For a person with Addiction, the pursuit of reward is not just driven by the availability of the substance or problem behaviours that produce a rewarding brain response. The pursuit of reward is also driven by intense memories of past experiences. This is coupled with apparent amnesia or minimization of past negative consequence and an obsession that is focused on seeking, finding, and using a specific behaviour or substance to stimulate brain reward circuitry to the exclusion of other behavioural options that could be available to the individual. Behaviour becomes all about acting out to an extent where motivation, willpower, and attempts at control will have limited or no impact. This is because the disease is in a high degree of activation, not because the person is weak. This is especially true in young adults who, in addition to having the disease of Addiction, do not have a fully developed frontal lobe, which is the centre of forethought, insight, and consequential reasoning. Therefore, attempts to increase motivation, willpower, and better choices will have limited benefit if implemented in a vacuum. These techniques can only be effective in the context of abstinence from all mood-altering substances combined with holistic recovery.

What is clear from research is that Addiction is about the brain and how interactions among reward, motivation, memory, and various frontal lobe circuits become translated into amplified 'go' responses and diminished 'don't go' responses.[15] Think of a traffic light; the non-Addiction brain has a clear red, green, and yellow light system to moderate behaviour. When one sits down to eat a meal, the green light says 'Go! I am hungry.' Part way through the meal, the yellow light comes on. 'Hey, let's slow down. I am starting to get full.' Soon after, with food left on the plate, the red light says 'Stop! I am full and do not need to continue eating.' In the brain of a person with Addiction, sitting down to the same meal, the green light comes on and says, 'Yes! I am starving, keep eating, do not stop, I need more.' The yellow light may come on later in the meal, 'This is not feeling great now, my stomach is nauseous' but the green light persists and overrides this feeling. 'It is okay, keep going, I need more.' The yellow and red light functioning is drastically impaired and will become progressively impacted as the disease continues over time. The person with Addiction will keep eating that meal until it is all gone or they are physically ill and cannot eat any more. It may not necessarily start off this way; some censorship and ability to say 'no' exists early on in the disease but, as time goes on, the yellow and red light falter more often. While the person struggling with Addiction knows that what they are doing is not healthy and does not feel good, the brain tells them to keep going. This is why, by the time people have come for treatment, providers will hear the common message, 'I don't even like using anymore; I just do it to feel normal.'

Thus, Addiction is not just about drugs, alcohol, or other sources of reward or relief that become a pathological pursuit in people who manifest the disease called Addiction. The 'go' is rationalized at times as a better choice than 'don't go' for the individual, even though it may neither be a choice, because of the compulsion involved in the disease, nor be rational as viewed by others. Therefore, Addiction is not solely about drugs, alcohol, or compulsive behaviours with gambling, eating, or sexual acting out; rather, these are symptoms of the disease that affects the brain. Attempts at behavioural control and management in treatment will be futile if the underlying cognitive, emotional, social, and spiritual components of the disease are not addressed.

CHAPTER SUMMARY

In this chapter, we explored how addictive behaviour encompasses the impact of alcohol, drugs, and compulsive behaviours in Addiction and recovery, as well as the role of prescription medications. We talked about some specific issues related to specific substances and behaviours but it is important to appreciate that the central drive to escape or avoid reality is the common reward pathway regardless of what the most effective reward may be for an individual. Complications that occur vary depending on the substances and behaviours that are part of an individual's manifestation of Addiction.

It is essential to assess relationships in every individual from the perspectives of a relationship with oneself, others, and a higher power to determine dysfunction. Assertiveness and boundary issues need to be explored during treatment on an ongoing basis to ensure that there is a healthy balance between meeting one's own needs and honoring the needs of others in a mutually supportive, interdependent manner. This is opposed to demanding or controlling behaviours filled with manipulation and resentments related to the unmet expectations that characterize dysfunction. We discussed the vulnerability to become stuck in the victim-perpetrator-rescuer triangle and, in recovery, the need to focus on being a survivor-helper-supporter.

Environment, exposure, and stress are three major pathways to relapse and addictive behaviour and have been built into the ASAM definition of Addiction. If one, two, or all three of these factors is present in the person life at any given time, their vulnerability for addictive thinking, and spiritual, emotional, cognitive, social, and behavioural relapse increases.

Chapter 6: Holistic Recovery: A Bio-Psycho-Social-Spiritual Perspective

This chapter focuses on the important components of recovery including self-management, and peer and professional support. We explore healthy behaviours in recovery from a holistic bio-psycho-social-spiritual perspective. We discuss goal setting and willingness, and the essentials of continuing care with Addiction as a chronic, lifelong disease. Lastly, we discuss post-acute withdrawal syndrome (PAWS), associated symptoms, and how long they can persist.

Addiction professionals and people in recovery know the hope that can be found through sobriety, which is the combination of abstinence and recovery. Recovery is available even to people who may not be able to perceive this hope, as well as to people who do not have Addiction. Anyone can benefit from the process of recovery. It can fuel fear, vulnerability, and angst amongst those contemplating or engaging in it. However, it is also a process that can propel freedom, serenity, relief, connection, and authenticity. Here we will explore the important components of recovery, its relationship with behaviour, and treatment from a holistic perspective.

COMPONENTS OF RECOVERY

As in other health conditions, self-management with mutual support is important in recovery from Addiction. Peer support, such as that found in community-based programs, whether that be 12-step groups (Alcoholics Anonymous, Narcotics Anonymous, etc.), SMART Recovery or others, is beneficial in optimizing health status and functional outcomes. Recovery from Addiction is best achieved through a combination of self-management, mutual support, and professional care provided by trained and certified professionals.

Self-management. Self-management involves employing strategies from the bio-psycho-social-spiritual model of recovery that one can implement in their own life. These strategies are diverse and some will work better than others for each individual. Thus, recovery is at times an experimental process as you find the activities and strategies that work best. Individuals with Addiction entering recovery often express a strong desire to 'do it myself' and believe that a high amount of motivation, willpower, and determination will carry them to recovery. Unfortunately, this is not the case as these are evidence of control tactics that feed the disease. The addictive mind tries to rationalize why you can do it on your own in a thousand and one different ways, when the reality is simple: self-management strategies alone do not work. They need to be used in the context of support, both peer and professional, with a focus on the whole being—physical, emotional, social, and spiritual. One has to be careful that the term self-management is not interpreted as being in control, rather it means identifying the process one needs to follow to deal with the disease.

Peer support. Peer support is essential for long-term recovery. Peer support can come from existing friends or family in the person in recovery's life, but often there are challenges to this. Sometimes existing friends or family members were using buddies, so even being around these individuals can increase vulnerability and risk of relapse. Sometimes existing friends or family members may be unhealthy themselves and struggle with the same disease of Addiction. If this is the case, the support that the person entering recovery needs will not be available from them. Thus enters another option: peer support coming from new friends, namely others in recovery.

The benefit of surrounding oneself with peers in recovery is powerful. These are people who do not just smile and nod when they are hearing stories about revelations, accomplishments, and personal growths that the person in recovery is experiencing. They feel true joy for the recovering addict, as they have experienced these joys themselves or are on the path to. Peers in recovery are also able to listen to struggles, cravings, relationship issues, frustrations, and feelings that come up with an authentic reality that others who do not struggle with Addiction or have not acknowledged their Addiction cannot. Here the person in recovery finds love and acceptance that they may not have experienced before.

12-Step Programs. Alcoholics Anonymous[1] (AA) is the original 12-step program, founded in 1935 by Bill Wilson and Dr. Robert Smith. After prohibition, Addiction (or alcoholism as it was narrowly looked at then) was perceived as a weakness, character defect, or moral failing that had no cure. There were limited treatment options available to those struggling, hence the creation of a peer-support program by Bill W. and Dr. Bob. While Addiction was primarily perceived as a personal failing and choice, there were those at the time, including one of Bill W.'s treating practitioners, Dr. William Silkworth, who believed it was more than that. Dr. Silkworth believed that alcoholism came with mental obsession and 'allergy' towards alcohol. His perspective was more accurately aligned with what is known about Addiction today. This idea positioned it as an illness, rather than bad people making bad choices. In addition to his theory about alcoholism, he also indicated that abstinence was necessary in order for recovery to be possible.

Bill W.'s treatment by Dr. Silkworth, as well as his time spent with a Christian fellowship called the Oxford Group, were built into the Alcoholics Anonymous 'big book', and became the foundation for the twelve steps. Since the inception of AA in 1935, the 12-step fellowship has blossomed around the world and developed groups that focus on substances or behaviours in addition to alcohol, including narcotics (NA); gambling (GA); overeating (OA); codependency

(CoDA); sex and love (SA, SAA, SLAA); anorexia and bulimia (ABA); and emotions (EA). There are also groups for family members of people with Addiction, such as Al-Anon, Nar-Anon, and Gam-Anon. Another 12-step group called All Addicts Anonymous (AAA) also exists but has yet to develop a strong or consistent fellowship in the world, although this program would be most in alignment with Addiction is Addiction.

All of these programs are free (although voluntary contributions to sustain activities are encouraged for those that can afford), community based, volunteer led and managed, and available all around the world. While 12-step groups may not be sufficient for the entirety of treatment for people struggling with Addiction (meaning that additional tools, groups, treatment, or resources will likely be necessary), they are certainly a valuable resource that is available most places at most times, making it one of the most accessible recovery support options in the world.

Many people struggle with the idea of attending these programs, particularly if they have not been to one before or have preconceived notions about it, including the spirituality aspect. While many describe these groups as religious programs, this is a fallacy. The 12-step programs contain valuable spiritual principles that transcend religious belief. Addiction is a self-centred, isolating disease, so the steps are designed to have one look beyond one's self and connect with something greater. This can be nature, other people, the universe, energy, the solar system, or anything you understand it to be; it does not have to be God.

From a holistic recovery perspective, this process provides growth in the emotional-social-spiritual realms. From an emotional perspective, it allows one to explore what it means to have a primary, chronic disease; the implications and consequence of the disease on self and others; the character traits that need to be worked on for a healthy self; and having a place (whether in meetings, reaching out to people in the program or working individually with a sponsor) to talk openly about feelings and experiences with people who understand. You cannot put a price on the value of being heard and feeling understood. Socially, these meetings allow people to connect with other people who have Addiction and are in recovery, which can be safer than associating with people who are active in their Addiction or do not understand the disease because they do not have it ('normies'). This does not mean your social network has to only consist of people in recovery, but it is important to keep in mind that people outside of recovery may not understand everything you have to say or be able to relate to your experience. For that, you may need to turn to people who also have the disease. Finally, spiritually, there is immense opportunity within the 12-step program to explore yourself, your internal spirit, and self-worth, and begin reaching out to others through amends and service work.

These programs are undoubtedly the most effective ways to achieve and maintain sobriety. This is likely due to their capacity to promote love for one's self and others, and to foster joy. The social component of the program contributes to these benefits, but it is also from the spiritual connection that is developed while attending meetings and working the steps. In fact, the founders of Alcoholics Anonymous intuitively and practically knew that the spiritual foundation was so essential that it was built into the first three steps of the program.

While there have been other support groups that have sprung up over time designed to be alternatives or complements to the 12-step programs, they have yet to develop strong fellowships.

Professional support. In recent times, the primary professional treatment intervention for Addiction has been psychosocial, sometimes called 'psychosocial rehabilitation'. It is usually provided by counsellors who may have training in the fields of social work and/ or psychology. Nursing and specialized physician support is also available in some outpatient or residential treatment programs. This treatment usually emphasizes the tenets and benefits of participating in ongoing peer support as well, such as through non-professionally-led community-based groups.

Various specific psychotherapies have been added to traditional recovery-oriented groups that emphasize abstinence as the foundation of recovery, including cognitive-behavioural therapy, motivational enhancement therapy, contingency management, network therapy, acceptance commitment therapy, and dialectical behavioural therapy. While the psychological (or emotional) and social components of the disease of Addiction are crucial to explore for healthy recovery, this model neglects the importance of care of the physical self and, most importantly, the spiritual self. There is an overwhelming resistance and reluctance amongst health care providers to bring up the topic of spirituality,[2] yet it is a critical foundation for healthy recovery, as evidenced by the 12-step programs.

It is important to find a health care provider, or team of practitioners, who are educated and knowledgeable about the disease of Addiction and can support the person in recovery through the holistic process of recovery. Objective outsiders are able to hear the disease in action more clearly than the addicted mind, but even peer supports can be trapped by the allure of addictive thinking. This is also how health care providers can be helpful as they provide an objective and neutral environment to hear and observe recovery and disease in action, which can then be discussed with clients.

Chapter 8 further outlines for health care providers how they can best support and provide treatment to people with Addiction, whether they have the disease themselves or not. This is a valuable addition to the treatment repertoire but, unfortunately, is not available to everyone desiring to get well due to financial or community resource constraints. Even if professional support is minimal or unavailable, there are still a lot of other recovery actions that can be taken by an individual to move them forward on their path.

BIO-PSYCHO-SOCIAL-SPIRITUAL DIMENSIONS

Individuals entering recovery have come to a place of realization that what they are doing is no longer working. Some hit 'rock bottom', which means appreciating that the consequences have become serious enough to take action; while others may not have had tremendous consequences from their Addiction but recognize the unmanageability and powerlessness of the disease. At this point, drugs are ingested because they 'have to be', not necessarily because they are wanted; hours spent on the casino floor now feel dreadful; and the physical, emotional, and relational highs and lows of Addiction have become tortuous. As Addiction has been the reality for so long, the process and promises of recovery seem vague, unclear, and overwhelming. Through education, time, awareness, and action, the unique process of recovery will begin to unfold at the level of alignment of values and meaning in life (spiritual), clarifying thinking and feeling distortions (psychological), developing a new, supportive social network (social), and attention to physical health (biological) with healthy eating and exercise.

HOLISTIC RECOVERY

Considering Addiction as a bio-psycho-social-spiritual disease, which has primary, neurobiological underpinnings, can explain the observable, wide-ranging behavioural manifestations of the condition. It is also a useful approach for recovery. Just as the disease of Addiction manifests differently in everyone, with some common traits underlying, so the process of recovery unfolds in a unique and individualized way, with some basic principles in common. Therefore, having a program that every individual is expected to fit into is often not an effective recovery approach and can lead to frustration for both the patient and health care provider's perspective. Having a thorough assessment to determine the individual's needs is a critical step in the treatment process. It is also important to learn about the bio-psycho-social-spiritual model of holistic recovery to personally or professionally apply it. Thus, individuals learn to tailor their recovery program to themselves with a combination of help from professional treatment and non-professional mutual support. It must be appreciated that all aspects of the disease need to be explored rather than focusing on just one substance or overt behaviour problem. Similarly, the 12-steps program needs to be personalized by the individual to themselves rather than blindly following someone else's program.

Biological. The biological, or physical, aspect of holistic recovery is the most accessible and familiar. Time spent in active Addiction, whether with alcohol, drugs, or problem behaviours, tends to wreak havoc on the body and can cause varying degrees of damage. Some entering recovery will have come out relatively unscathed and may exhibit signs such as loss of muscle tone, elevated cholesterol, or weight loss. Others entering recovery will have more severe physical complications, such as cirrhosis of the liver, hepatitis, or damage to internal organs.

When entering recovery, it is important to be thoroughly examined by a physician, preferably one who is experienced in Addiction Medicine. For many people with Addiction, it has been years since they have had a regular physical check-up because of fear and shame related to what complications may be developing. Having an examination can provide a starting point to see if regular medical care and treatment is necessary. If this is not done, recovery work may be hampered by ongoing physical symptoms that have not been attended to. For example, pain from a physical health issue contributes to frustration and lack of energy. These feelings then become attributed to the process of recovery not working and make it challenging to follow through on healthy activities.

Other aspects of physical health include diet and exercise. Nutritionally valuable foods are important to consume, especially while the body is recalibrating without substances or problem behaviours to soothe it. Hydration with water helps flush the system and eating regularly throughout the day stabilizes blood sugar and metabolic processes. Regular physical activity (20 minutes, 3-4 times per week) provides routine and structure to recovery in addition to the health benefits it provides, including lowered cholesterol, maintenance of healthy weight, muscle strengthening, and cardio-vascular benefits. For those who are reluctant to engage in exercise, walking around the block or neighbourhood is a great place to start.

Psychological/Emotional. The reality of 'feeling the feelings' is no easy proposition to someone entering recovery. After all, these are the feelings that the addictive process has escaped, avoided, and sought relief from. The concept of Pandora's Box often comes up when talking to patients in early recovery or contemplating recovery. Patients worry that if this box is opened, a flood of feelings will come flowing out that they are incapable of dealing with or processing in a healthy way. Fear takes over. This can lead to avoidance, attempts at control, and the worst possible outcome: relapse. It is important to appreciate that fear is just a feeling, though an uncomfortable one, that will pass, as all feelings do. The challenge is to identify that fear and other feelings are present and work with them, rather than avoid. This is what the addictive process is all about. The recovery challenge is to look honestly at feelings and recognize them as mes-sages. For instance, fear is the body's way of saying that attention needs to be paid to a situation. It is providing awareness of a real or perceived threat to wellbeing. Avoidance or escape from this message could have severe consequences to one's health.

This is true of all feelings across the spectrum. If one can learn to allow feelings to flow, much like the current in a stream, rather than jump into the river and try to control the flow of the current or run away from the stream all together, life will feel profoundly different and more rewarding. Listen to the messages: What is anger trying to say? What information is boredom providing? What is joy telling you? Feelings are an invaluable guide to navigating the self and situ-ations. They provide information about the world and the self's place within it.

As feelings arise, one can write, paint, talk, and explore them. Over time, the person in recovery will find their personal and unique ways to deal with feelings using a variety of techniques. This is an entirely new world for some, as often those struggling with

Addiction come from homes in which feelings were not acknowledged, let alone talked about or shared, which contributes to the anxiety and angst one feels in doing this for the first time. This too is a feeling that will pass, if you let it. Identifying and processing feelings, however, is something that people can learn over time if they are open and willing. In recovery, people will notice that they transition from their primary feelings being fear, anger, and shame, to having faith, acceptance, and serenity. Recovery provides a toolbox for ways to deal with the emotional turmoil and pain on a difficult day, and to staying in reality without needing to escape them.

The psychological aspect of recovery attends to feelings and brings in a focus on self-talk–the ongoing, internal dialogue that affects how people feel and behave. This was discussed in depth in the Addictive Feeling chapter. Increased awareness of self-talk can expose the vulnerability of the disease, including the shame, anger, and fear that fuel low self-worth. Rather than thinking 'I did bad' (guilt), the addictive mind translates this into 'I *am* bad' (shame). Shame-based thinking feeds fear-based thinking. If one feels unworthy, there is the perceived risk of rejection or abandonment by others. The threat of exposure of an authentic or real self is terrifying to someone struggling with shame 'because there is no way a person will like what they see. I don't like what I see.' The internal dialogue centers around this: 'I'm stupid; people hate me, why would anyone love me?' Anger grows as self-hatred grows, 'How could I be so stupid? Of course I'm unlovable, look at me.' These feelings are fuelled by shame and fear.

This is how self-talk is used by Addiction for its own selfish gain. People who feel shame, fear, and anger seek escape or relief from these feelings, sending them right back into the throws of their Addiction. However, on the recovery side of the street, self-talk can be a tool of empowerment. Being more gracious and kind in the inner dialogue is the beginning of a relationship with self. Rather than old patterns of thinking fed by shame, fear, and anger, one can consciously work on new ways of thinking. Instead of the focus on what one is not doing or what is not working, internal dialogue focuses on gratitude, acceptance, and surrender of imperfections, as in these examples.

> *"I didn't do that perfectly but that's okay. I handled it the best I could with where I was at in that moment."*

> *"I might feel like a screw up right now, but I know I have a lot to offer others and myself."*

> *"I'm annoyed that driver cut me off. Maybe they are having a tough day."*

Empathy and compassion, not just for others but also for oneself, builds as internal dialogue is explored. If people are interested in consciously working with their self-talk, it is helpful to begin by developing awareness. Writing down common thoughts is a starting point, as there are so many thoughts running through our minds each day that are not noticed, though they will still have an impact on feelings and behaviour. After doing some writing and listening to your thinking, it is time to start exploring different ways to talk to yourself, as we have discussed previously in Chapters 3, 4, and 5. Consciously introduce more grace and compassion into your thinking and be mindful of the traps set out by thinking, like the 'woulda, coulda, shouldas' or 'why?' questions.

Addictive thinking can be difficult, if not impossible, for a person in recovery to hear within themselves. While self-management tools, like self-talk, are helpful, they cannot be used in isolation. It is essential that people in recovery journal their thoughts and feelings and 'check it out' with others. It is only when addictive thoughts are concretized in writing and vocalized that they can become obvious to the person in recovery, but also to those who are listening, who can then provide valuable feedback. Becoming aware of addictive thinking can promote further recovery action and slow the momentum of the disease.

Social. The social aspect of recovery revolves around relationships, old and new. Some people will naturally drift out of life, some will be actively detached from us because they fuel vulnerability, and others will come into life as a gift of recovery.

As the mind clears in recovery, existing relationships often feel different. Take Peter as an example. Peter numbed himself since the age of twelve with marijuana, tobacco, and later on alcohol, consuming up to thirty-five beers per day by the age of twenty-nine. When Peter engaged in the recovery process, he became distraught. Daily living, which included taking care of a home, wife, and children, became overwhelming. Being asked to discipline his son for not cleaning his room became a major stressor that he felt incapable of dealing with sober. After multiple relapses, Peter decided to accept his family's invitation for residential treatment, where he could focus on his personal journey of recovery outside of his daily environment. Household squabbles that he detached from during active Addiction presented a reality that was uncomfortable to Peter. Over time, he learned to communicate effectively, set appropriate boundaries, and engage in self-care when feelings were coming up for him. Dealing with conflict and the possibility that people may get upset is particularly challenging in recovery, as this challenges the image management and relationship parts of the disease that call for civility regardless of what is happening and the desire to maintain peace at all costs.

In recovery, the dysfunction of family members may become apparent. It is discomforting to see sickness in loved ones, as they have often been placed on a pedestal. Families can create a dynamic in which the visibly active person with Addiction is the 'sick one' and everybody else is a witness, not an active participant in the disease. The focus is on the identified patient and desperate calls for treatment and support are pushed toward this individual. This dynamic of 'us' versus 'them' becomes routine in the family and when the identified 'problem' person begins to get well, this creates a significant shift for the others. Now attention and energy is freed up that allows family members to reflect on themselves and, more often than not, they realize that they have also been part of the problem through enabling, poor communication, inconsistent boundaries, or minimization. The feelings that arise from these realities are challenging, but also offer profound opportunities for growth.

Reality shifts in recovery. More accurately, reality is not shifting so much as the *perception* of it. The people, places, and things the person in recovery thought they knew and understood change as they gain clarity, and this is often where the appreciation of a need to make both minor and major changes in lifestyle arise. Kate, mother of two, struggled with sobriety throughout her life. However, once she was able to establish a few months of abstinence through attending meetings, seeking therapy, and journaling, she started to gain some clarity and realized that her teenage daughters were trapped in their own disease. They created drama and chaos with each other and her, which made it challenging for Kate to maintain recovery action. Only when she was able to step back from these relationships, disconnect with love for a while, and focus on her, were the promises of recovery able to blossom in her life. This was Kate's challenge. For others it might be relationships, past trauma, shame, or the desire for control that are barriers to recovery. As one begins the process of recovery, the personal barriers will become clear, with the help of peer and professional support, and one will be able to devise a recovery plan that allows them to deal with these challenges in a healthy way.

Spiritual. The role of spirituality in recovery is often not a standard part of residential or outpatient treatment programs. 'I don't believe in that religious stuff,' or, 'I'm not religious so I don't want to talk about it,' or, 'I've never even thought about that and am not about to start now,' are some examples of resistance when spirituality is brought up in a professional recovery context. Often spirituality becomes likened to or synonymous with religion, which is a sensitive topic for many people, particularly if they have been raised in a religious environment or have a challenging relationship with it. Religion is designed to be a spiritual source of comfort and advice. It provides a structure of moral guidelines and a community for those in need. But it is not for everybody. Spirituality is the discovery of our authentic self without any trimmings or labels and is available to everyone. Spirituality gifts us with a rich source of values and a deeper meaning to life. Religion can be a means to an end in spirituality, but it is not a necessary means. Spirituality, however, is essential in order for the person in recovery to get well.

Within recovery, spirituality connects the person struggling with Addiction with a love outside of themselves, being their higher power (HP) of choice. Feeling unconditional love and understanding that one is not alone are powerful antidotes to the feelings of abandonment, loneliness, self-hatred, and shame that stem from the disease of Addiction. Connecting with an HP through meditation, prayer, time in nature, reflection, reading, or journaling fosters a sense of serenity, peacefulness, and calm that can be helpful when cravings and uncomfortable feelings surface. As recovery progresses and the relationship strengthens, it becomes the foundation for long-term abstinence and leads to the promises of recovery.

Addiction is often described as a selfish disease. Certainly when people are entrenched in it the focus is on self—more specifically, the self's quest for escape, relief, and reward through substance or problem behaviours. Recovery can be misperceived as selfish, but more accurately, the recovery process is self-focused, not selfish. A gift of recovery is the ability to share one's love and personal attributes with others because life is no longer driven by the quest for escape, but rather in finding pleasure in all the things life has to offer, including relationships. A spiritual foundation shifts the focus from 'I' to 'other' as one starts to see life outside of one's self. Beginning to see an HP and its role in life connects one to the reality that there are others out there, which breaks the mind, soul, and spirit free from the trap of Addiction that says 'It is all about me.'

Spirituality, believing in a force other than oneself, and connecting with this, brings with it feelings of hope, faith, gratitude, and serenity. Hope is the feeling that what is wanted can be had or that events will turn out for the best. Hope is different than expectation, where one is looking for a particular outcome. Hope is trusting that your HP and recovery will move things forward in the way that they need to, not necessarily always in the way one may want it to. When one is tied to specific expectations about how events, conversations, or relationships will develop, they are already setting themselves up for resentment. For example, someone who is attending a work conference on communication who expects to have lots of opportunity to hear about the various types of communication and see demonstrations of what those look like may become very disappointed and resentful when the majority of the conference is exercises and role playing. While this was not what the person expected, perhaps this is what they needed. If they are not open to this process, however, they will hang on to that resentment and describe that conference as 'useless.'

Expectations are often called 'premeditated resentments.' Faith is part of the process of healing, allowing us to move freely through our lives. It can be overwhelming to trust the universe's plan and relinquish control and expectation, but it is necessary for serenity, acceptance and true freedom. Faith is the antidote to fear. Fear is often internally created and is fed by the expectations that are being carried about people, places, and things. Fear can keep one paralyzed and stuck in wondering 'what if'. 'Can I trust this person? What if they betray me?' 'Can I succeed in recovery? What if I relapse?' Hope and faith can break the chains of fear and allow one to live in the moment and accept any possible outcome, recognizing that they are neither 'good' nor 'bad', but what needs to be at that moment. For example, if that person does betray you, were they somebody that you needed to have in your life anyway if that is their approach to relationships? Often relapses can teach valuable lessons and provide great amounts of clarity, though they are scary and difficult to go through. Ability to accept these messages can often lead to a sense of gratitude. Even when outcomes are uncomfortable and it may be difficult to see the higher power's plan in them, one can be thankful and ready to show appreciation for the guidance. With hope, faith, and gratitude comes a sense of serenity; a beautiful feeling of tranquility in which the mind, body, and soul are quiet and calm. The mind stops racing with 'what ifs' and trying to control or predict outcomes. Rather, it is taking in the information being provided and letting it go.

No one would turn down the opportunity to experience hope, faith, gratitude, and serenity. Unless, of course, they were trapped by a disease that feeds them misinformation: 'Those feelings are bogus, they are not even possible and certainly not real, especially for you as you do not deserve to feel anything good.' This is the trap of Addiction. Spirituality is part of the path to freedom from these traps of shame and self-loathing.

Within Addiction, spirituality is commonly the most underdeveloped aspect of self and the first to take a backseat when relapse vulnerability builds. Meditation, prayer, journaling, and reflection begin to wane as the disease waxes. This is more reason for spirituality to be a focal point in recovery, as it provides valuable information as to the state of the disease. If spirituality is strong, disease vulnerability is lowered. If spirituality is shaky, disease vulnerability is higher.

Powerlessness. When the 12-step programs were developed in the mid-twentieth century, the founders intuitively and practically understood that surrendering in relation to the disease of Addiction and acknowledging both *powerlessness* and *unmanageability* were the necessary first steps to getting well. Hence, step one explicitly states, "We admitted that we were powerless over [our Addiction] and that our lives had become unmanageable." What makes the process of surrender so important? The disease of Addiction is all about control. The disease feeds the mind information that 'If I try harder, do better, am more motivated, things will be okay.' This is the starting point of shame because, of course, the disease is uncontrollable once it has been activated, until a person can recognize the role of the disease in their life and choose recovery. Only when the illusion of control has been let go can the process of recovery unfold.

BEING AND DOING (IN RECOVERY)

Activities in holistic recovery include taking care of the body, mind and spirit. Not all of the activities possible in recovery will work for everyone, but developing a toolbox of recovery is important. Gone are the days of relying on one go-to escape, reward, or relief mechanism, which is what Addiction is all about. What will work for self-care and nurturing today may not help as much tomorrow, but that does not mean it is not a helpful tool to keep in the toolbox. Thankfully, there are other tools that can be tried out when the hammer is not enough.

One challenge that arises throughout the recovery process is accepting life on life's terms. A mind struggling with the disease of Addiction believes in the predictability and ability to control life. If a situation does not seem to be going the way it was planned, the addicted mind fights against this tooth and nail. Futile attempts at control take up time, energy, and headspace, which is detrimental to the recovery process. Acceptance of the unpredictable nature of life begins to take shape in recovery.

Acceptance and connectedness with everything allows one to experience being rather than just remaining attached to or focused on doing. The doing is a means, a process, whereas the being is the end experience.

RECOVERY PLAN

It is essential to have a recovery plan as a proactive method to guide your daily activities rather than trying to do things on the fly. It is important to have moments to just 'be' as well as to 'do' in life and recovery. Thankfully, recovery action can help one become more comfortable with being in recovery.

To help you build your own personal recovery plan, review the following list and check off the activities you are already doing or aspire to.

Table 2. Recovery Activities Checklist

☐ Drink lots of water

☐ Eat nutritiously

☐ Meditate

☐ Journal

☐ Draw, paint, create

☐ Song, poetry writing

☐ Assertiveness

☐ Hobbies (sports, crafts, music, book club, other)

☐ 12-step meetings

☐ Community meetings (e.g., SMART Recovery)

☐ Say no

☐ Let go

☐ Prayer

☐ Disconnect from unhealthy people

☐ Set boundaries

☐ Identify my needs

☐ Exercise 3-5 times per week

☐ Equine therapy

☐ Reaching out to friends, family and healthy supports

☐ Individual therapy

☐ Group therapy

☐ Feel the feelings

☐ Mindfulness

☐ Deep breathing

☐ Abstinence from mood altering substances

☐ Admitting powerlessness

☐ Learn more about Addiction

☐ Meeting with clergy/spiritual leaders

☐ Hypnotherapy

☐ Acupuncture, other complementary treatments

☐ Signing up for retreats, activities

☐ Accept

☐ Go to church

☐ Yoga

☐ Have fun!

Appendices E and F are also designed to help support you in your recovery journey. Appendix E is a sample recovery schedule that shows how it is possible to incorporate recovery into life and not the other way around (where recovery takes priority). Appendix F is a blank template for you to use in creating your own schedule. Routine and regularity are important in recovery because this helps stop the disease from taking you for a ride.

GOAL SETTING

In active Addiction, goals and priorities become skewed. A helpful tool for goal setting is to use the SMART[3] approach. This means making goals: Specific, measurable, attainable, realistic, and time-specific. Exploring ways to set realistic, healthy goals in recovery is an important part of the lifestyle shift. Firstly, the more specific and clear a goal is, the more likely it is to be attained. For example, the vague goal of 'I want to be healthy' becomes 'I am going to start walking twenty minutes per day, three times per week.' This way the goal becomes more tangible and measurable. At the end of the week, one can ask, 'Did I reach my goal of walking three times this week?' If yes, congratulations! If not, what can be done differently this upcoming week? Writing the goal down in a calendar, committing to another person for accountability, or planning a specific time to do the walking is also helpful.

If the goal continues to be challenging to meet, the automatic feeling is shame, followed by the thought, 'I am not trying hard enough and this is not working. I give up.' Rather than give up, perhaps the goal needs to be re-evaluated. Commit to walking two times per week rather than three and see how this goes. It is important to be realistic in the recovery goal-setting process, especially if you are prone to perfectionism and taking on too much. The perfectionist tendency with Addiction pushes one to strive for unattainable goals like to do 'recovery right and right now.' It is important to focus on progress, not perfection.

It is important that goals be realistic, but also slightly out of one's comfort zone such that they encourage growth and development. For example, for someone who has never exercised before and commits to four workouts per week, this may be overwhelming. The more unrealistic a goal, the less likely it is to be accomplished. Rather, starting with one or two workouts per week may be more manageable. Ideally, goals are things a person wants to do. Otherwise, motivation will be low. This comes up often with 12-step meetings; people do not know what they will get out of it so the mind says it is not desired. However, if the individual has a desire to get well and enter recovery, this would be an action to take as it may help move towards this overarching goal.

Other tips with goal-setting include: Making them measureable and able to be tracked so one can congratulate themselves and see progress; have a timeframe attached so the goal does not get lost in the hurriedness of life; be specific; and write down the goal and steps to accomplishing it. Write down appointments, commitments to yourself with eating, the gym, meetings, etc. Often people get into trouble with goals because they are too unrealistic or lofty, they are looking for an instant reward, and do not establish accountability so goals get lost in the disease. The challenge with Addiction is that the mind tells you that a goal needs to be big and it needs to be attained now, otherwise it is not worth it. These are the all-or-nothing, grandiosity, and instant gratification aspects of the disease in action.

In recovery, the challenge is to set realistic goals and be mindful that instant reward is not always likely and goals will take time not only to achieve, but also to feel the benefit from. Simplifying intentions can help slow down the mind when it begins to feel chaotic. Particularly in early recovery, focus on the immediate needs and priorities rather than being caught in futurizing, which is where obsession and compulsion can arise. As with all parts of the recovery process, take goals one day and one moment at a time. There is no benefit to having the mind set up camp in the past or future; here and now is where life is.

When working on recovery and life goals, appreciating and congratulating you for steps forward is an integral part of the process, even if what has been done seems insignificant. These are all meaningful and important steps that have often not been taken before. Appreciation and gratitude can help with continued motivation and goal setting. The whole process may feel uncomfortable, overwhelming, and new, which is to be anticipated, but this does not mean recovery does not work or is a bad thing.

The process of recovery is likely both more and less obvious now. If you are struggling with Addiction, clarity may be building on what you would like to do, but roadblocks may be popping up telling you these are not things you need to do. It is important to appreciate that the latter message is likely being fed by the disease and is false information. If your intuition is screaming that you need recovery, than that is the voice of the authentic self. As a health care provider or family member watching others struggle with Addiction, it may be hard to internalize the magnitude and power of the recovery process. There will be a temptation to become caught up in focusing on behaviour, rather than appreciate the thinking, feeling, and being parts of the disease. Given time, patience, and practice, clarity can and will develop. However, the process of recovery can only begin once the first step has been taken by the person struggling with Addiction, and that is the step of willingness.

WILLINGNESS

All of the recovery actions discussed above are well intentioned and can produce phenomenal results, but only once a willingness to change has been reached. For some this willingness comes when they hit rock bottom, meaning the lowest point in one's Addiction. Job loss, marital breakdown, children being apprehended by child services, near-death experiences, bankruptcy, and homelessness are all stark examples of the depths this disease can take one to. Not everyone reaches a bottom like this before entering recovery, and not everyone who reaches this kind of bottom proceeds to develop the willingness to get well. Willingness is an individual process and looks different for everyone. Whenever and wherever the willingness begins is also where the shift begins from active disease to recovery.

It is essential that the stages of change[4] be kept in mind during assessment and treatment so individuals can be approached at their own place in their development. Change is thought to occur in five stages: precontemplation, contemplation, preparation, action, and maintenance. Each of these helps in understanding how ready somebody is to make a change in their life. For example, someone who is in the precontemplation stage is displaying resistance and may say things like 'Get off my back, I'm fine.' The person in precontemplation is often unaware that there is a problem and has yet to come close to a rock bottom. During treatment with someone who is in precontemplation, the focus needs to be on developing rapport, gathering information, and expressing concern regarding what is being observed rather than focusing on goals and giving action steps for them to complete.

Once there is some evidence that the individual is aware there is a problem but may still be somewhat ambivalent, this is the contemplation stage. You may hear people saying things like 'I am not sure I can do it, but I would like to.' At this stage, it is important to gather information and provide guidance to prepare for change, rather than trying to convince. Doing so can spark fear, resentment, and defensiveness and push the individual back to a precontemplation stage. Discussions involving the pros and cons of making a change become important at this stage as this discussion can help elicit clarity from the individual of what is and is not working in their life. Attention is often needed on the cons of making a change (fears, roadblocks) and the pros of not making a change (or staying as is) to address what is keeping people trapped. Discussing the cons of staying the same (or consequences of their actions) and pros of making change are rather obvious and are likely already being considered by the individual.

When there is a movement towards 'I want to change, who can help?' the care providers can become more directive with suggestions. This is the preparation stage in which individuals are open to change but may not know what to do. It is important to capitalize on this sometimes narrow window of opportunity and provide the individual with multiple options for their health, including outpatient and residential treatment options. There is a high risk at the preparation phase that individuals will lose momentum and slip back to contemplation or precontemplation stages. If this happens, it is important not to get discouraged. If someone has reached the preparation stage before, they can get there again.

When you hear, 'I need to change and this is what I have been doing. What else can I do?' this is someone in the action phase. They may have already started taking steps to change their current situation and have a high level of motivation and momentum. At this stage it is important to emphasize that 'Alone one can't, but together we can.' It is important that people be using supports around them, both formal treatment as well as informal peer, family, and friend support, to maintain the momentum.

The maintenance stage is where people have been involved in action to change their lives. It takes 2-5 years of action before one can be considered to be in the maintenance stage, which is where the new way of living in recovery feels more familiar. This way of life is now more sustainable and natural, with less effort required to maintain it. It is essential during the maintenance stage that one watches for stressors or complacency, as these can take an individual back into contemplation and relapse very quickly. Resistance, especially internally, is part of the recovery process and it is important that individuals, family members, friends, and care providers deal with the resistance without going into fear, anger, shame, or resentment. The table below summarizes the stages of change, what those changes look like, and recommendations for how to support people at each of those points.

Table 3. Stages of Change

Stage of Change	Experience	Recommendations
Pre-contemplation	What problem? Ambivalent	Start listening to those around you and be open to their feedback. They may be able to see what is going on better than you can
Contemplation	Maybe there are problems?	Take a look at what is going on and start to consider the problem and changes that need to be made
Preparation	Who can help me? Preparing to move forward	Seeking out resources, materials, people and support to help
Action	Doing and following a plan	Staying connected and engaged in treatment path
Maintenance	Recovery feels more natural	Recovery actions are integrated as priority and life fits around them

ESSENTIALS OF CONTINUING CARE FOR LIFELONG RECOVERY

Recovery is an ongoing process and does not stop, even if certain milestones are met, such as completing a residential treatment program or being abstinent for five years. This is the reason we refer to recovery as continuing care rather than 'aftercare,' which is a term used by many. The question becomes 'after what?' whereas continuing care reinforces the need for an ongoing consideration of health. It is important to remember that all treatment interventions are part of continuing care and the recovery process, none are better or worse than others, and all aid in growth.

In active disease, individuals undergo frequent intoxication and withdrawal. There are symptoms, signs, and complications associated with specific substances and behaviours that need to be recognized during the initial assessment so that if physical dependence is present, appropriate recommendations can be made for a safe withdrawal management process. Recurrent withdrawal is a powerful driver of continued engagement in substance use and addictive behaviours to seek relief (which is negative reinforcement). This may occur when what may have been rewarding in the past no longer provides any positive reinforcement or reward. Substances may damage organ systems; hence, a routine part of assessment and treatment monitoring needs to include biological indices, such as measuring liver profile, kidney function, hematological indices, and thyroid function. This needs to be done together with a physical examination by a physician, focused specifically on gathering evidence of damage to the body organ systems.

In some instances, such as for nicotine or opioids, agonist maintenance therapy may be considered for a short or long duration. Agonist maintenance therapy is sometimes called replacement or substitution therapy and involves treatments like nicotine gum or patches, or methadone or Suboxone. Specific issues in the treatment for each substance or addictive behaviour need to be taken into account, which is why it is important to understand the main manifestations of the disease and speak of 'Addiction involving' without getting caught up in compartmentalizing each symptom as separate. Continuing care needs to be interdisciplinary so that the strengths of training backgrounds of each team member, including physicians, social workers, psychologists, nurses, counselors, etc., are included and all treatment providers operate under a common framework in a complementary fashion rather than as individuals just adding their perspectives.

Treatment for Addiction needs to devote specific attention to substances such as alcohol, nicotine, opioids, and behaviours, such as binge eating, purging, or other complications, which can affect physiology, specific organ systems, and overall health status. However, more specific attention to craving, cue response, preoccupation, impaired control, and the balance between 'go' (pursuit of reward) and 'don't go' (healthy inhibition or modification of such drives) would be needed to ensure that the commonalities related to the persistence and progression of active disease are better appreciated. Treatment also needs to devote attention in its psychoeducational content and cognitive-behavioural interventions to how impairment of control can increase the affected individual's vulnerability to preoccupation, craving, and a pathological relationship with a range of potential sources of reward or relief.

Social and peer support are essential as well. The 12-step programs continue to be a cornerstone for fellowship and recovery structure; however, they are presently divided in terms of substances and other behaviours. The establishment of Narcotics Anonymous became necessary more than half a century ago because Alcoholics Anonymous groups were unwelcoming to people with heroin as their drug of choice. Over the years, Overeaters Anonymous, Gamblers Anonymous, Cocaine Anonymous, Sexaholics Anonymous, and Sex and Love Addicts Anonymous have been established for social and spiritual support. Even today, some people who may be abstinent from using alcohol and be a long-term member of AA continue to act out in Addiction with food, sex, or gambling without full awareness that their disease is still active. There is an essential need for continuing care that would be mindful of and monitor all aspects of Addiction treatment and recovery.

POST-ACUTE WITHDRAWAL SYNDROME (PAWS)

By definition, PAWS[5] is a series of persistent symptoms that may occur long after stopping substance use, while one is in recovery from dependence on benzodiazepines, barbiturates, alcohol, opiates, antidepressants, and other substances. Symptoms of PAWS include mood swings resembling an affective disorder; anhedonia, which is the inability to feel pleasure from anything beyond use of the drug; insomnia; extreme drug craving and obsession; anxiety and panic attacks; depression; suicidal ideation and suicide; and cognitive impairment such as difficulty making decisions, poor memory, and lack of attention.

PAWS is post-withdrawal syndrome or protracted withdrawal syndrome. It affects many aspects of recovery and everyday life, including the ability to keep a job and interact with family and friends. Symptoms occur in over 90% of people withdrawing from long-term opioid use such as heroin, 75% of people recovering from long-term use of alcohol, methamphetamine, or benzodiazepines, and to a lesser degree from other psychotropic drugs. Post-acute withdrawal syndrome from benzodiazepines, barbiturates, alcohol, and opioids can last from a year to several decades or indefinitely, with the symptoms entering into periods of relative remission between periods of instability. Benzodiazepines are the most notable drug for inducing prolonged withdrawal effects with symptoms sometimes persisting for years after cessation of use. Severe anxiety and depression are commonly induced by sustained harmful use of alcohol, which in most cases abates with prolonged abstinence. Even sustained moderate alcohol use may increase anxiety and depression levels in some individuals. In most cases, these drug-induced symptoms fade away with consistent, prolonged abstinence. It is extremely important to recognize that the physical withdrawal symptoms can be triggered by external environmental cues and internal mood states in individuals who have Addiction. The chronic nature of this disease, in context of the memory circuitry being affected, means that there is no time limit over which PAWS is totally in the past. Individuals in treatment need to become aware and remain vigilant about their own particular triggers that reactivate PAWS and may create a relapse risk. Dealing with feelings and life stressors effectively and honestly are necessary aspects of preventing and coping with PAWS. Withdrawal symptoms abate in a supportive, caring environment; hence, it is necessary for people in recovery to have a circle of people to reach out to on a regular basis to prevent PAWS and mitigate the symptoms if triggered by people, places or things.

CHAPTER SUMMARY

As with other chronic health problems, self-management combined with mutual support is important in recovery from Addiction. Recovery is best achieved through a combination of self-management, mutual support, and professional care provided by trained and certified professionals. Considering the bio-psycho-social-spiritual aspects of the disease of Addiction is also necessary for recovery. Just as the disease of Addiction manifests differently in everyone, with some common traits and underpinnings, so the process of recovery unfolds in a unique and individualized way. A bio-psycho-social-spiritual framework of holistic recovery optimizes outcomes. It is essential to have a recovery plan to proactively guide daily activities rather than trying to do things on the fly. Part of the recovery plan is to set realistic, healthy goals as a necessary part of the lifestyle shift. This whole process of recovery can only begin once the first step of willingness has been taken.

Addiction, being a chronic disease, requires continuing care utilizing professional and non-professional resources. Professionally facilitated continuing care needs to be mindful of monitoring all aspects of Addiction including symptoms of post-acute-withdrawal syndrome (PAWS), which can affect many aspects of recovery and everyday life. Withdrawal is a powerful driver of continued engagement in substance use and addictive behaviours to seek relief from discomfort, also known as negative reinforcement, even under circumstances in which what may have been rewarding in the past no longer provides positive reinforcement.

Chapter 7: Family Members

This chapter is for family members and highlights that Addiction's impact extends well beyond the individual with this disease. Addiction is considered a family disease and everyone in the family plays a role. Healthy boundaries, communication, self-care, and emotional healing are discussed in more detail to help family members live a more balanced and healthy life.

Addiction is a disease present in an individual but it extends to all family members and relationships. With active Addiction, all family members are impacted adversely and all family members need to be in recovery for themselves. It is common for family members to see the person with Addiction as the problem and, as such, they are often unaware how they aggravate the disease. To best help your loved one with recovery, it is essential that all family members understand Addiction as a chronic brain disease. Without this understanding, it is difficult to change family patterns and move forward with healthy recovery. It is common for family members to become preoccupied and consumed with the person with Addiction such that they start to lose sight of their own needs and neglect their own self-care. With active Addiction, relationships within the family become increasingly dysfunctional. There is no healthy balance between meeting one's needs and honoring the needs of family members in a mutually supportive, interdependent manner. Rather, the relationship tends to become demanding or controlling, filled with manipulation, distrust, expectations, and resentments that are related to the unmet expectations on all sides.

In family therapy, the whole family is the patient, with individuals being subsets of the entire whole. Family therapy within the context of Addiction is used to work towards a family life that is substance-free, and reduce the impact of Addiction on the family and individuals within the family unit. In consideration of this, various forms of family therapy are now incorporated into intensive outpatient and residential treatment programs. It is also common for family members, including spouses, parents, siblings, and children, to attend individual therapy appointments with the individual with Addiction to address issues of communication, boundaries, and behaviour, known as family-involved therapy. If treatment is only geared towards the person with Addiction, who then returns to a family environment filled with dysfunction and challenges, this will pose many problems for recovery and increase the risk for relapse. Therefore, it is important that family members be involved in the recovery process in terms of education and action around their own self-care and health.

The relationship with a significant other or spouse is also important to address in the context of recovery. Avoidance of fantasy and projection is necessary to ensure that social interactions and relationships are grounded in the reality of 'what is' as opposed to 'what should be.' Humans are social creatures and relationships are an integral part of our experience. Everyone has support needs that can be achieved in healthy relationships that foster personal growth and self-esteem. Healthy relationships allow people to be accepted for who they are when there is reciprocity and respect between the individuals. Reciprocal relationships require a spirit of cooperation, as well as an understanding of and ability to embrace interdependence. Interdependence in a healthy relationship requires that both people accept personal responsibility. One person cannot take all the blame while the other person gives it all. Relationship dynamics that foster caretaking or dependence in the context of unreasonable demands or abdication of responsibility inherently aggravate Addiction.

In recovery, it is essential to move beyond codependence or Addiction involving relationships to interdependence for all family members. Acceptance of responsibility for the creation of a reciprocal relationship takes a high degree of emotional maturity, personal awareness, and time to develop. Interdependence is the key to any healthy relationship and can be defined as staying true to one self, having boundaries that are firm yet flexible, and knowing when and how to give help—but also knowing when to say no. It is about caring and giving to others but doing so with consciousness and compassion (not martyrdom), and with enough self-awareness of when to pull back before it negatively affects your own health and wellbeing.

FAMILY ROLES

In families with Addiction, family members often take on certain roles as a by-product of living with active Addiction. Unless family members seek help and recognize the dysfunctional role that they are playing in the disease, problems worsen and all family members are negatively impacted. Here we will explore the common roles that family members take on when there is Addiction in the family. These can apply to children, siblings, relatives, or spouses of people with Addiction. These roles[1] are the person with Addiction, chief enabler, hero, scapegoat, mascot, and lost child.

The *person(s) with Addiction* in the family is/are likely experiencing a high amount of pain and shame, although they may not be aware of this as the result of substance use or acting out. As the Addiction progresses, the person with the disease is faced with increasing feelings of shame, guilt, inadequacy, fear, and loneliness, and develops a number of defenses to hide their shame and guilt. These may include irrational anger, charm, rigidity, perfectionism, social withdrawal, or hostility. Anxiety, panic attacks, or depression can also become a cover. The person with Addiction often projects blame or responsibility for their problems onto other things or other people, including family members, who also take on unhealthy roles in order to survive within the chaotic family unit. It is for such a person to be labelled as selfish or a narcissist but those labels are not helpful. The grandiosity of a person with Addiction, making themselves to be bigger than they are in reality, is reflective of the shame generated by the disease and the lengths to which the affected person goes to keep it hidden, either consciously and sub-consciously. Family members need to be aware that their efforts to point out problems may actually exacerbate shame and accomplish the opposite, which is to have the person with Addiction become more defensive or avoidant.

The *chief enabler* or *caretaker* typically steps in and takes control while the person with Addiction is active in their disease. Their purpose is to maintain appropriate appearances to the outside world. Enabling is anything that protects the person with Addiction from the consequences of their own actions. Spouses often take on the role, but children and siblings can also be enablers. The intent of enabling is to solve specific problems with the belief it will help, yet they end up perpetuating or exacerbating current issues. An example is a family member who purchases alcohol for their loved one with known Addiction. The family member may rationalize this purchase with the belief that 'at least the person with Addiction will not have to drink and drive and will, therefore, be safe.'

Another example of unhealthy enabling behaviour is a family member volunteering to call the employer of their loved one with a feigned illness when, in fact, they cannot go to work because of a hangover. While well intentioned, the enabling behaviour serves to protect the person with Addiction from taking accountability and responsibility of their recovery and consequences related to the disease. The enabler tends to everybody's needs in the family and by doing so, becomes out of touch with themselves and their own needs. The caretaker is often so busy that they do not take time to assess their own needs and feelings and, therefore, develop the insight needed to make changes within the family unit. As long as the enabler and the person with Addiction play the game of mutual self-deception, health for all parties will only decline.

The *hero* in the family is the high achiever. Their purpose is to raise the esteem of the family. They are the person who takes the focus off the person with Addiction because of their success and accomplishments. They can be perfectionists, feel inadequate unless they succeed, be compulsive, and become a workaholic later in life, though this can be evident in school-age years as well. Often the hero is the oldest child, who may see more of the family's situation and feels responsible for fixing it. This child typically excels in academics, athletics, music, or theatre and gets their self-worth from being special and successful. The hero does not receive attention for anything besides achievement; therefore, their inner needs are not met. As things get worse, the hero is driven to higher levels of achievement, propelled by the false belief that this will fix their internal pain and external chaos. However, no level of super-responsible, perfectionist, over-achievement can remove the hero's internalized feelings of inadequacy, pain, and confusion. The hero often ends up distancing themselves from the family of origin and many grow up to marry people with Addiction and become enablers, a role they are familiar with; or they may manifest more overt active Addiction later in life.

The *scapegoat* or *rebel* is the family member that goes against rules, acts out to take the focus off the person with Addiction, and feels a tremendous amount of hurt and guilt. Often because of their behaviour, they can bring help to the family because they are the lightning rod for family pain and stress. Often the message to this individual is that they are responsible for the family's chaos, when actually the misbehaviour of the scapegoat serves to distract and provide some relief from the stress of Addiction within the family. The scapegoat typically has issues with authority figures as well as negative consequences with the law, school, and home. On the inside, the child is a mass of frozen feelings of anger and pain and may show self-pity, strong identification with peer values, defiance, and hostility, or even suicidal gestures. This role may seem strange in purpose. However, if there was no scapegoat, all other roles would dismantle. S/he allows others a pretense of control and the person with Addiction is not identified as an issue, as often the scapegoat is identified as the problem, often with active Addiction in them.

The *mascot/cheerleader/clown* uses humour to lighten difficult family situations. They often feel fear, others see them as being immature, and they are limited to bringing humour to all situations, even when not appropriate. This individual is typically the most popular in the family as they bring fun, humour, and a sense of lightness into the family unit. The clown enjoys getting attention and making people laugh, especially when the anger and tension of substance use are dangerously high. These individuals are often named a class clown in school. They frequently demonstrate poor timing for their comic relief and most people do not take this child seriously. They are often hyperactive, charmers, or cute outwardly but inside, they feel lonely knowing no one really knows the real person behind the clown's mask. The clown may grow up being unable to express deep feelings of compassion and put themselves down often to cover up their pain with humour. The mascot's purpose is to provide levity to the family, and to relieve stress and tension by distracting everyone.

The *lost child or wallflower* is typically withdrawn and a loner with little or no connection to the family. S/he brings relief by not bringing attention to the family and they have difficulty learning communication and relationship skills. The lost child has much in common with the scapegoat, as neither feels important and they see much more than is vocalized. The lost child often builds a quiet life on the outskirts of the family and is seldom considered in family decisions. They hide their hurt and pain by losing themselves in the solitary world of short-term pleasure, which may include excessive TV, reading, listening to music, drugs, object love, eating, and fantasy. The favorite places for the lost child are in front of the TV or in his/her room, and due to the sedentary lifestyle, a lost child is vulnerable to issues with weight. As adults, they feel confused and inadequate in relationships and may end up as quiet loners with a host of secondary issues such as sexuality problems, weight problems, excessive materialism, or heavy involvement in fantasy, which all adds up to Addiction even if excessive substance use is not part of the picture. The lost child usually does not place added demands on the family system as he/she is considered low maintenance in younger years, and often labelled a 'lost cause' later.

Families fall into these roles regardless of how far the Addiction has progressed along the continuum. Often the roles that people identify with will change over time, such that you may identify with a few of the roles rather than just one. These roles may become more entrenched as the disease progresses, but characteristics and traits will be obvious from early on, even when the Addiction's severity is less. As the family unit lives in these roles, relationships within it disintegrate and members will admit that none are entirely comfortable in the role they have unknowingly stepped into. As external circumstances change, the family is less able to adapt. If a crisis or alteration in the system occurs, such as a death, birth, or divorce, the roles simply switch to accommodate the change. For example, a child may have been a lost child in their younger years while living in the family unit, but grow up to be a mascot in college.

The examples listed above are not exhaustive but help to demonstrate some common roles within a family that occur to cope with stress associated with the disease. To move away from these, it is essential that each family member, including those with Addiction, take responsibility for their own health and healing and enter recovery. Steps to doing this include gaining awareness of the role you have played in your family and what your vulnerabilities are (e.g., rescuing, people pleasing, avoiding, minimizing, and so forth). Additional steps beyond awareness include developing, establishing, and maintaining healthy boundaries; doing your own emotional processing and healing; communicating assertively; and developing and implementing your own healthy recovery plan, using the holistic bio-psycho-social-spiritual framework.

HEALTHY BOUNDARIES

Al-Anon, the 12-step program providing support to individuals who have family members with Addiction, endorses the '3-C rule': 'You did not *cause* it, you cannot *control* it, and you cannot *cure* it.' Many people, even when recognizing the disease, feel they are responsible for another person's Addiction. They try to control it and hang on to a false belief that they can cure it. This leads to misery and frustration for everyone. This is a false sense of control, for only the individual with Addiction can take accountability and responsibility for their recovery.

Boundaries[2] are, therefore, an essential part of recovery for people with Addiction and family members alike. In a nutshell, boundaries are guidelines, rules, or limits that a person creates to identify what are reasonable, safe, and permissible ways to interact with other people around us and how the person will respond when someone pushes those limits. Boundaries are set by you, for you, and are about what you will and will not accept for yourself. People often mistake boundaries for external limits that once set, other people have to respect and enforce. However, boundaries are always internal, meaning that they are set and enforced by the individual, for the individual. They require assertiveness in action, which is taken by the individual for personal safety and sanity rather than expecting or demanding the other person to change.

For example, you decide that your boundary is that you need personal space on Thursday afternoons and your partner does not pick up the children from school, as mutually agreed upon. It would be your responsibility because it is your boundary, not your partner's, to have a backup plan and arrange for a friend's parent or other family member to go and pick up the kids so that you can still have your self-care time. The tendency for some, however, would be to resentfully give up their self-care time, pick up the kids, and spend time with them until your partner comes home when you passively, aggressively, or passive-aggressively lash out for them not picking up the kids. This would be an example of inconsistent boundary setting in which actions are not congruent with words. Making alternate arrangements displays congruency, or being true to your words through actions. This is what boundaries are.

In healthy recovery where there are boundaries, the individual with Addiction stops people pleasing and making other people happy to make up for their past transgressions and make other people happy. Helpers and family members stop trying to fix, persuade, problem-solve, or rescue, and focus on their own health and well-being, providing support that is reasonable to them if and when their family member is accepting and open to this support. One example is driving them to a 12-step meeting or counselling therapy because they have scheduled the appointment and agreed to go. Rescuing, which is swooping in to problem-solve and fix any issues that may come up, is a form of control that can feel like persecution to the person with Addiction, leading to increased shame and resistance to change. The irony in families is that members are typically well-meaning, yet can often end up driving disease activity through their rescuing tactics, which come with the indirect, and unintentional, message of 'You are not (doing) good enough.' Once boundaries are put in place, there is greater distance and objectivity for everyone to see clearly what needs to be and what can be done, rather than becoming entangled in the person and situation such that clarity becomes sullied.

Boundaries require an appreciation that another person cannot do for someone what (s)he needs to do for themselves. One has to move beyond codependence or Addiction involving relationships to interdependence, which means supporting each other to develop one's own identity, with mutual support, relying on each other as helpers and protectors, in terms of reality checks and accountability.

To develop and enforce boundaries, clarity around the question of 'who am I?' and healthy communication are essential.

EMOTIONAL HEALING

The healing process for family members is just as important as for those with the disease of Addiction. There are many feelings generated for family members of people with Addiction, including fear, resentment, anger, guilt, and shame. It is important to be mindful of all feelings that come up and to not judge them or label them as good or bad. Feelings provide us with valuable information that is necessary to listen to in order to heal emotionally and be on the path to health.

Fear. Addiction is a scary disease and can lead to premature death if left untreated. Everyone knows this part of Addiction, even if the rest of it is somewhat of an enigma. Therefore, fear is a natural response for any family member who sees their loved one being led down the garden path into the weeds by their Addiction. With this realization comes a sense of powerlessness. Emotionally you know that there is nothing you can do—this disease will take your family member where it will regardless of what you say or do—yet the mind may at times convince you that you *do* have the ability to change the course of what you are seeing. This is where control comes from, which can also be labelled rescuing, caretaking, or problem solving. Everyone, including the person with Addiction, knows that these behaviours are well intentioned and come from a well-meaning, caring place. Let us be clear, though—they do not work. Living in fear and letting this drive controlling behaviours generates resentment, guilt, and shame that only serve to feed the disease and do not reinforce recovery for anybody.

Resentment. For family members who do not have the disease of Addiction, it is difficult to understand what their loved one is going through. They cannot understand the cognitive dissonance, shame, and self-hatred; all they can see are promises not being lived up to, actions not being taken, continued failures at sobriety, and a wave of destruction being cast down on the family unit. When this is all they see, it is not surprising that resentments build. Family members will often say they are 'just trying to survive' and keep functioning in their own lives and activities, though inevitably having to deviate from these plans to compensate for Addiction in the family. This puts family members in survival mode, where they do what needs to be done to survive, but the opportunity to thrive does not exist. Thriving means to have the time and space to explore themselves, interests, feelings, and develop the self beyond the levels of feeding, clothing, and cleaning. As they focus on survival, they stew and resent, often casting blame on their family member, not just the Addiction, for having put them in this predicament. Many family members believe that having their loved one enter recovery is the only way to move beyond this state of being, as well as move beyond their resentments. However, it is possible for family members to enter recovery before their family members do. Everything that is discussed in this chapter, including healthy boundaries, emotional processing, identifying values and meaning, and healthy communication, are part of breaking this cycle and moving from a state of surviving to thriving.

Letting go of expectations. This is the key to letting go of resentments. If people carry the expectation of an outcome (e.g., 'That if my husband goes to residential treatment our life will be so much better when he returns,' or 'If my wife would only drink less, we would be happy,' or 'My recovery will cause my brother to see the light and get well too'), then they are setting themselves up for disappointment and resentment. People can have hope that things will change, but hopes are fluid, flexible, and adapt as the process unfolds. Expectations are rigid, inflexible, and defined so that if anything does not go according to plan along the way, the reaction is to become resentful. Letting go of expectations means staying in the process and being open to whatever outcome may happen, even if it was not one you could foresee but trusting it will be what you need, not necessarily what you thought you wanted.

Anger. When people carry resentments, which come from expectations, they are also carrying anger. For family members, anger can be directed inwards, outwards, or both. Any way you look at it, this anger is a destructive force in the health and happiness of the individual. As discussed in previous chapters, with anger it is essential to go below the surface and explore what is truly happening at the emotional level. What this means is that anger is a composite emotion, comprised of many feelings that have been building up for some time until they merge and come out as anger. Therefore, when you are reacting with anger about your loved one coming in late, not putting away dishes, or not paying the utility bill, you are reacting to that event as well as many others that have gone unprocessed. Family members of people with Addiction are often shocked at the uncharacteristic anger that can begin to become a regular, almost routine, part of their lives. This is often because they are focusing on maintaining the family flow (i.e., surviving) rather than exploring their own health and recovery.

Guilt and Shame. As discussed in Chapter 4, related to addictive feelings, it is important to distinguish between guilt and shame because people often confuse the two when, in fact, they are different experiences. Guilt is a thinking process about action: 'I did bad.' Whereas shame is carried at such a deep emotional level people may not even know that it is there, which makes it challenging to bring to the level of awareness. Shame says, 'I am bad' and is just as destructive to the health and wellbeing of family members as it is to people with Addiction, though the behavioural consequences of not addressing shame can be bigger for those with Addiction (e.g., relapse or acting out which can lead to death, jail, or institutionalization).

What do family members carry guilt about? Potentially everything: 'Do I need to do more to help? Did I do too much? How did I let it get here? If only I had... If only I could... Should I have done that? Was that too harsh? Am I doing enough? How can I focus on me at a time like this?' Active Addiction is a minefield with the potential for guilt cropping up around every corner, though the early days of recovery may not feel that much better. As mentioned above, it is important that family members enter their own recovery even if their loved one with Addiction is not ready to, but this can also come with a heap of guilt, loaded on from within and without. Taking care of one's self will inevitably shift the established dynamic in the family and household. When people are unstable, they react unpredictably, so family members entering recovery can initially seem to add to the turmoil, though inevitably this is necessary and in everyone's best interests.

Bring shame into the emotional landscape and things can seem even more complicated, as family members may want to get well themselves, or even leave the household. If they are carrying too much shame, this becomes an impediment because the shame tells them, 'You don't deserve better, this is all that there is for you so suck it up and deal' or 'What kind of person leaves their sick family member?' However, if your family member is not willing to work on recovery than this may be a necessary option for your health and safety, as well as theirs. Shame casts doubt on ourselves, our actions, and purpose, and can make things muddled, to the point that people give in and continue to live in survival mode because they do not see any other deserved option. This, of course, is not the case. Everyone on the planet is worthy of safety, comfort, and health, but shame can disfigure this fact.

ACTION

Awareness of each of these feelings and how they affect you is an important step in the recovery process. This can be done through talking with supports or a therapist trained in Addiction. Other helpful activities include journaling, prayer, meditation, reflection, and body scanning to learn more about these feelings. It is also important to begin to explore the question of 'who am I?'

Who Am I? Identifying values, meaning, identity, and purpose. When people enter recovery, whether you are the family member of a loved one or the person with Addiction, usually a lot of time and energy has gone into surviving daily life. The focus is largely external, whether on another person as in the case of family members, or substances or problem behaviours in the case of people with Addiction. During this process, less time, attention, and energy is put into connecting with your true sense of self and really understanding what you value and enjoy. Therefore, the overarching existential question of 'who am I?' looms for anyone entering recovery and can feel daunting and overwhelming. While it may *feel* bad, remember that nothing is ever bad in itself. It is our perceptions that can trap us or motivate us to change. All things in life provide opportunities for growth.

Reconnecting with or recovering who you are is no easy task and can be facilitated by asking yourself the following questions:

- What are my core values? (Examples may include determination, honesty, integrity, loyalty)

- What do I enjoy doing and find fun?

- What recharges me? (For instance, does quiet time or doing something with one or two close friends provide you with an influx of energy, or does being engaged in a group activity or lively discussion leave you feeling invigorated?)

- What do I feel is my purpose on earth? What would I like to contribute to myself and others?

- What do I feel passionate about or have felt passionate about in the past?

- What am I looking for in a healthy relationship with myself and others?

You may need to spend time over many months, or even longer, talking through and writing out your answers to these questions. The process of disconnecting from yourself took time, so reconnection cannot happen instantly—but will come quicker than you anticipate.

Strengths/affirmations. With an increase in shame and disconnection from self comes a decrease in self-esteem, confidence, and self-worth. Rediscovering and eventually liking and loving yourself are essential for lifelong health and wellbeing. Active Addiction can come with a lot of mean words and hurtful statements that slowly erode one's appreciation and compassion for self. Recovery for family members involves identifying traits and characteristics that you embody and learn to appreciate. A simple but powerful way to do this is through affirmations. They provide emotional support and encouragement to one's self. They may be read online, through quotation books, or created by you, for you. For best results, it is important to practice affirmations regularly throughout the day because you may have unconsciously developed the habit of negative, destructive self-talk. It will take some time, but is possible to override this with healthy self-talk. The more conscious time and effort you can put into affirmations and focusing on strength, the more natural this process will become.

To create affirmations, make a list of traits and characteristics you demonstrate. These can be traits you are aware of or things others have told you about yourself. All you need to do is add 'I am' to the beginning of these traits and they become affirmations. For example:

I am... *strong*

I am... *worthy*

I am... *capable*

I am... *content*

I am... *resourceful*

I am... accepting

I am... compassionate

I am... genuine

Depending on where you are in your healing journey, having these affirmations become internal truths may seem like a long way off, but it is amazing how resilient our subconscious and unconscious minds are. Carrying one of these affirmations in your mind each day and repeating them as often as you can does have benefit and will not take as long as you think to become more natural.

As your sense of self strengthens and recovery progresses, you may notice a shift in your communication or, if you are early on in your recovery, you may want to take purposeful action to change your communication from unhealthy to healthy patterns. This can benefit everyone in the relationship, not just family members.

HEALTHY COMMUNICATION

As you grow and reconnect with who you are, you will start to clarify the needs and desires that previously you either did not share or that were not being met in your current relationship. Once you embrace your own recovery path, however, you will start to see the need to communicate your needs and boundaries appropriately to others. Communication, both verbal and non-verbal, is an essential ingredient for any healthy relationship and can change along with awareness and action.

Non-verbal communication. When the term communication is used, most of us automatically think of talking, or verbal communication. People forget that there is so much more to communication, particularly the non-verbal elements,[3] including body language and listening.

Body language sets the stage for a conversation. For healthy communication to occur, it is important to convey that you are open, engaged, and in the moment with the other person(s), all of which are demonstrated through our non-verbal body language. Healthy communication is open, whereas many disconnections in communication can happen when body language, and therefore communication, is closed.

Table 4. Body Language

Open Body Language	**Closed Body Language**
Facing the other person	Body facing away from the other person
Looking at the other person, making some eye contact that is comfortable to you	Looking at the ground, around the room, or anywhere but at the other person
Arms unfolded, hands in lap or at sides	Arms crossed, folded over the chest
Leaning slightly towards the other person	Leaning back, away from the other person
Using some hand gestures to be congruent with your words	Staying unmoving, stoic and not having your body match what you are saying
Remain relaxed, comfortable	Present as tense, uptight, or defensive

It is also important that the tone of voice remains calm, evenly paced, and clear while one is practicing open body language so that the two are congruent. When your body is aligned with what you are saying and how you are saying it, the meaning of your message will be clearer. When there is communication breakdown, something goes awry at one or all of these levels. Communication breakdown may involve muttering, yelling, trailing off before a sentence is finished, talking too quickly, and the closed body language signs described above. Even if the message is being articulated verbally, the meaning and impact may be lost as it comes out.

As the listener, it is easy to get caught up in our own thinking and to plan a response to what the other person is sharing. If you find yourself doing this often, beware, as you may not be hearing people properly. When people are consumed by their own thoughts, they are not fully present and, therefore, not hearing everything that the other person is trying to convey. It can be challenging to stay present and engaged, particularly when the situation is emotionally sensitive or triggering, but it will help keep the conversation on track. Truly listening, not pretending to (as many people do), involves hearing every word that comes out of the other person's mouth, pausing to reflect on what they have said, and paraphrasing what you heard to ensure you are accurate in your interpretation. Let us explore an example:

> *Ray (the person with Addiction): "I need you to under-stand that when you are calling and texting me mul-tiple times per day to find out where I am and what I'm doing, it frustrates me. I feel like a child who cannot be trusted to be on their own and I'm resentful. I know you are trying to help me but it doesn't help!"*

> *Sandra (family member, who is not listening): "Resentment?! You want to talk about resentment?! How do you think I feel not knowing where you are, what you're doing, when you'll come home, or if you'll come home at all? It's terrifying! Remember two years ago when you disappeared for two days? I can't go through that again Ray! Do you think I like having to keep tabs on you? Of course not but I'm so scared I don't know what else to do."*

> Ray: "Geez Sandra, you just don't get it! I'm pouring my heart out here and all you can do is criticize me! Don't you think I already feel like garbage enough?"
>
> Sandra: "Oh Ray, what do you want me to say? What do you want me to do? Nothing helps, nothing works."

In this example, Sandra was caught up in her emotional reaction to what Ray was saying. Therefore, her response was to one of his words, resentment, and she reflected her own struggles with that to Ray. In these cases, communication is already at a standstill, even if people keep talking, because now they are caught up in a defensive/offensive conversation. Let us explore what it would look like if Sandra was truly listening to Ray.

> Ray: "I need you to understand that when you are calling and texting me multiple times per day to find out where I am and what I'm doing, that it frustrates me. I feel like a child who cannot be trusted to be on their own and I grow resentful. I know you are trying to help me but it doesn't help!"
>
> Sandra pauses to reflect on what Ray has just said. "I hear that I'm treating you like a child and you don't want to be around me when I'm doing that."
>
> Ray: "No, no. When you are checking up on me, it pushes my shame button and I feel unworthy. I feel more vulnerable to acting out because I can't stop reflecting on what a schmuck I am and how much pain I have caused to everyone around me. It's not that I don't want to be around you; I don't want to be in myself."
>
> Sandra: "Okay, so if I understand you, my calling and texting, which is driven by my own fears and

insecurities, drives you to feel more shameful and inse-
cure, which probably doesn't help with your recovery. I
just don't know what else to do, Ray."

Ray: "Well, obviously the calling and texting isn't
working. It sounds like it brings up just as much fear,
shame, and frustration for you as it does for me. I
know you are trying to be supportive of my health, and
I appreciate that, but there must be other ways for you
to support me that feel comfortable to both of us."

This dialogue becomes different from the previous one when empathy and paraphrasing are used. Stopping to reflect back what you are hearing to the other person and conveying understanding of their feelings are essential tools to an open dialogue. In this scenario, healthy action is already happening as both are expressing their feelings related to the calling and texting. As an added bonus, at the end of the conversation it looked like Ray and Sandra were at a point that they could start to look at alternatives that would be healthier for both of them. Again, this is a bonus, not the intention of the conversation. Ray's intention was to share his feelings. If you can be clear that expressing feelings is the goal of communication, things will flow more easily than if you are attached to a particular outcome or expectation for action.

Here is a reminder for healthy communication strategies when you are the listener:

Table 5. Effective Listening Strategies

Effective Listening

Hear every word that the other person is sharing

Do not think about what they are saying or plan your response as they are talking

Be present in the moment

Effective Listening

After they finish speaking, paraphrase or reflect back what you heard

Keep doing this until the speaker agrees, 'You have understood me'

Be empathic and understanding

If you have effective non-verbal communication skills, your words and message will be clearer.

Verbal communication. What is said is only a small part of effective communication, as the majority of our communication is actually non-verbal, but it is still an important thing to be mindful of and attentive to. It is especially so when trying to set boundaries or shift how you are engaging with people. While a lot of these boundaries and shifting in approach are apparent from our non-verbal communication, the message and words used are still part of the overall package.

The four styles of verbal communication[4] that are important to understand are:

- *Passive*: Those with a passive communication style are generally afraid of confrontation and do not feel they have the right to make their own wishes and desires known. They may be apologetic, deferential to others to make decisions, and do not assert their needs.

- *Aggressive*: Aggressive communication is a method of expressing needs and desires that does not take into account the welfare of others. The aggressive communicator may appear domineering or bullying, doing anything they can to get their way in a conversation.

- *Passive-Aggressive*: The pattern of behaviour wherein an individual swings between the passive and aggressive communication styles depending on the moment or situation. On the surface, he/she appears passive and indifferent but in reality acts out anger in a subtle or indirect way, often through sarcasm, condescension, or patronization.

• *Assertive*: Communication characterized by a confident declaration or affirmation of a statement without need of proof. This affirms the person's rights or point of view without being threatening or aggressive, nor tiptoeing around the issue. The assertive individual is confident, self-aware, believes in their value as well as others', decisive, proactive, and consistent. In communication, the assertive individual embodies the healthy non-verbal communication strategies reviewed earlier and is clear and direct in expressing their needs. You may hear the assertive person say, 'I choose to...'

To be assertive moves one towards healthy communication and relationships. It means that you are clear about who you are, what is important to you, and can clearly and simply articulate this to others. Getting to a place where you can be assertive can involve time and a lot of personal exploration and growth, particularly if you are entrenched in another way of being. However, all of the tools of recovery mentioned throughout this book will help move one towards assertiveness.

When you are assertive, boundaries can be more clearly identified, set, and followed through on. Assertiveness also means being able to say 'no' as a complete sentence. This means with no justification, explanation, or rationale required. This can happen if the same scenario keeps happening repeatedly as family members play out their old dysfunctional roles. This is particularly true and tough for family members who are vulnerable to people pleasing and not wanting to rock the boat. The three simple steps to saying 'no' are: (1) to open your mouth, (2) to say 'no', and (3) to close your mouth! The internal dialogue that can happen around how to say 'no' without upsetting the other can keep the mouth closed. For example, 'how do I tell my mother that I do not want to go to a party with her without hurting her feelings?' If the mouth is not closed as in step three, a story may follow to soften the 'no', which makes it more likely that the message will change from 'no' to 'maybe' to even 'okay'. There can be some waves generated in relationships as people explore new ways of communication and assert their needs but ultimately everyone benefits from this. If the people in your life cannot handle this way of being or respond poorly, this is confirmation that they are not healthy and do not need to be in your life anyway. If they are true supports and good relationships, then they will see that all of these changes are for the better and support you in your journey, even if it is uncomfortable to them at first.

CHAPTER SUMMARY

With active Addiction, all family members are impacted adversely and need to be in recovery for themselves, not just for the affected person. Recovery involves exploring health from all aspects and devoting time and energy to reconnecting with who you are, identifying strengths, having time for self-care, identifying and processing feelings, and communicating effectively and clearly with those around you.

In families with Addiction issues, members often take on certain roles as a by-product of living with active Addiction. Unless family members seek help and recognize the dysfunctional role that they are playing in the disease, problems worsen and everyone is negatively impacted. Part of being in recovery is learning to set healthy boundaries and appropriately communicate your needs with others in a healthy, respectful manner. Healthy communication requires a lot of practice and willingness on the part of all as the family unit adapts to a recovery style of living. At times, it may be important to draw clearer boundaries with 'No' as a complete sentence, without getting into story telling (excessively explaining the reasoning and hoping for understanding) or apologizing ('I am sorry but...'). The development of interdependence requires all family members to work through their own issues.

Chapter 8: Health Care Provider Roles and Responsibilities

This chapter is directed towards health care providers who need to learn more about the importance of assessment for Addiction, as its complications present so commonly in everyday practice, and tailored treatment for Addiction that is necessary for healthier outcomes. Details regarding assessment, as well as current issues in care, favoured treatment modalities, and barriers to treatment are discussed. We explore the importance of education and proper training for health care professionals and developing individualized treatment plans rather than adopting a 'one size fits all' model of care where the patient is expected to fit into a pre-designed program with little appreciation of individual differences.

IMPORTANCE OF ASSESSMENT AND TAILORING TREATMENT

The recognition that Addiction is a primary, chronic disease that has broad manifestations requires initial comprehensive assessment and ongoing care in a therapeutic environment. As the disease has been recognized to express itself along biological, psychological, social, and spiritual dimensions, assessment and treatment need to be developed and implemented along these lines as well.

The importance of a comprehensive assessment and treatment approach that allows tailoring the treatment to individual needs in a continuing care framework is vital. Thus, the treatment program needs to be adjusted on an ongoing basis within a chronic disease framework based on the readiness and willingness of the person rather than sending them to different short-term programs that may or may not meet all of their needs. For example, having people go for relapse prevention education followed by anger management group therapy followed by individual counselling that focuses on specific stressors. Rather, looking at the bigger picture of Addiction and ongoing activities people can engage in to address their physical, emotional, social, and spiritual health while getting consistent feedback and support would be preferred. The recommended components to setting up such a comprehensive assessment and treatment plan are discussed further below.

Clinical interventions can be quite effective in altering the course of Addiction even when the process is complicated and the desired outcomes elusive. It is essential to monitor closely the behaviours of the individual in the context of how various aspects of the disease are manifesting. Contingency management, sometimes including consequences for relapse behaviours, can contribute to positive clinical outcomes.[1] Engagement in health promotion activities that promote personal responsibility and accountability, connection with others, and personal growth, also contribute to recovery. It is important to recognize that Addiction can cause disability or premature death, especially when left untreated or treated inadequately. Therefore, it is important to appropriately screen and intervene, as Addiction issues are often not obvious or the presenting issue.

The qualitative ways in which the brain and behaviour respond to drug exposure and engagement in addictive behaviours are different at later stages of Addiction than in earlier ones, indicating progression, which may not be overtly apparent. As is the case with other chronic diseases, the condition must be monitored and managed over time to:

a. Decrease the frequency and intensity of relapses;

b. Sustain periods of remission; and

c. Optimize the person's level of functioning during periods of remission.

In some cases, medication management can improve treatment outcomes. Often, the integration of psycho-social-spiritual treatment and ongoing care with evidence-based pharmacological therapy provides the best results. Chronic disease management is important for minimization of episodes of relapse and their impact. Treatment of Addiction saves lives.

ISSUES IN ASSESSMENT

Considering Addiction as a single condition has profound implications for treatment, however, it is typically treated using separate programs for treatment for each manifestation, such as alcohol, drugs, sex, and gambling. For instance, drug addiction treatment, alcohol addiction treatment, and nicotine addiction treatment have evolved on vastly different tracks over the last fifty years. This has led to treatments with differing philosophies and theoretical models; different regulatory and funding streams; and even different ways of training professionals. As discussed in earlier chapters, it is important to not be caught up in what the person is 'addicted to', as this can miss the thinking, feeling, and spiritual implications of the disease. Rather, health care providers need to explore how the disease is manifesting, such as Addiction involving alcohol, tobacco, and gambling. This shift in language recognizes that there is much more going on than just the drinking, smoking, or gambling. While this may seem like an issue of semantics, the language used around Addiction is meaningful and has consequences in terms of how people approach treatment and recovery.

Historically, treatment for Addiction involving gambling has been accepted in some circles, while treatment for the other so-called 'process addictions' has been looked upon with more skepticism. The treatment of Addiction involving sexual issues, in particular, continues to face great scrutiny and stigma. Addiction involving sexual issues is often treated separately from other behavioural and substance issues, though the underlying process is the same, in separate treatment centres or separate programs within the same treatment centre as some theoretical models view this as a different kind of Addiction from all others.

A unified approach to Addiction treatment needs to be the common standard of care, together with follow-up in a chronic disease framework of ongoing, continuing care. In this treatment approach, the emphasis is on tailoring treatment to the individual and recognizing that Addiction is Addiction. This approach involves comprehensive treatment for a unitary disease with multiple manifestations that can be associated with any number of pathological sources of reward and relief. This simplifies treatment and recovery action for the person with the disease and allows multiple symptoms associated with the disease (e.g., depressed mood, physical withdrawal symptoms, communication issues, and isolation) to be treated at the same time. This is in contrast to previous formulations of the disease and its treatment, which tended to talk about 'addictions' requiring unique clinical approaches based on the specific source of reward (e.g., the specific class of drug, or the addictive behaviour). Even in the unified approach, unique pharmacological features of different addictive drugs and behaviours need to be appreciated to provide specific guidance and care for specific needs and complications tailored to the specific needs of the individual. However, the appreciation of commonalities allows for clarity in awareness related to what is required in treatment and recovery. As different pharmacotherapies target specific neurotransmitter pathways and receptor systems, the tailored approach can target different mechanisms of action of medications in specific circumstances.

This approach to treatment, which is aligned with the ASAM definition, attempts to find commonalities of clinical approaches and suggests concurrent attention to the multiple manifestations of Addiction, rather than a sequential approach in which patients are matched to different treatment approaches. As Addiction is about differences in the brain functioning of people with the disease, not necessarily about their specific behaviours, the stigma related to these, such as acting out with sex or drugs, can be transcended.

Many treatment programs presently exist that are designed around the experience and philosophies of their founders and treatment providers. The focus is often primarily on alcohol or other drugs only, and it is uncommon that a treatment centre insists on treating Addiction involving tobacco at the same time as drugs and alcohol. The so-called 'process addictions' are often not addressed or referral is made to a specialized program, such as for sex addiction or eating disorders, either before or after residential treatment for substance dependence or substance use disorder. Thus, the patient is matched to a pre-set program, presumably based on their identified need. The need itself is often self-identified or by an assessment that is focused primarily on the most problematic substance used in the patient's behavioural repertoire, rather than through a comprehensive assessment that includes exploration of all possible aspects of the disease, especially behaviours related to food and sex. Treatment matching may or may not include the use of medication(s) depending on the philosophies and policies of a particular program, rather than what the true needs of an individual patient may be. Discharge from the program is often called 'graduation' and variable amounts of 'aftercare' are recommended. All of this, sadly, perpetuates the acute care model of treatment that somehow people are fixed once they have achieved abstinence from specific substances or completed an intensive program.

The primary professional treatment intervention for Addiction has been psychosocial, sometimes called "psychosocial rehabilitation".[2] This approach uses a multidisciplinary team of clinicians, but centers around the work of the certified addiction counselor, who is usually not a physician, psychologist, or nurse. They are the primary clinician or case manager, and employ group, individual, and family therapy. This is widely known as professional addiction treatment in North America. This treatment usually emphasizes the tenets and benefits of participating in ongoing peer support, such as that available through non-professionally-led, community-based 12-step groups. Various specific psychotherapies such as cognitive-behavioural therapy (CBT), motivational enhancement therapy (MET), contingency management, network therapy, acceptance commitment therapy (ACT), 12-step facilitation (TSF), and dia-lectical behavioural therapy (DBT) have been added to traditional recovery-oriented groups that emphasize abstinence as the founda-tion of recovery. Each of these is a psychosocial intervention, most frequently administered by an addiction counselor, a social worker, or a psychologist with a wide variation in their training backgrounds.

The major issues within these traditional types of treatment is that often the main care providers, whether they are addiction counselors, other health care providers, or peer support group, do not have proper education or information on the disease from an Addiction Medicine perspective. It is easy to get trapped in a focus on behaviour management and focusing on abstinence with one or a few substances, which still leaves the individual sick and strug-gling with other aspects of the disease. It is important to know how Addiction is manifesting beyond substances in areas such as food, sex, relationships, gambling etc. as well as in feeling, thinking, being, spirituality, connection, memory, and communication; interven-tions must be targeted at all of these levels in addition to abstinence from using substances.

A comprehensive assessment includes taking a family and developmental history of the individual, a chronological history of substance use and engagement in any other addictive behaviours, and a history of other medical, psychiatric, or surgical problems or complications. The health record would also document issues along the biological, psychological, social, and spiritual dimensions to highlight the manifestations of the disease in those areas so that treatment interventions can be tailored effectively. For example, the genetic heritage, a physical examination, and bloodwork results would be essential components of the biological dimension. These are important for all new patients to complete, even if they do not have Addiction themselves, as there may be underlying vulnerabilities or conditions impacting their recovery. In some cases, people may be coming for help who do not believe they have Addiction as it is their family member who does, but in reality they have it too and this can sometimes be spotted through biological testing.

Problems related to thinking and feelings would be part of the psychological dimension of the evaluation. The social assessment would include exploring problems related to housing, income (work or disability), family, and friendship networks. Lastly, but importantly, the spiritual dimension would involve assessment of what gives meaning to the individual's life, what their important values are, the relevance of religion to them, and whether they have a personal connection to a higher power. Physician involvement is essential in this process, as it would be for any other disease or illness.

TREATMENT SETTING, INTENSITY, AND DURATION

Individualized treatment requires attention to the level of care a person may need, with regards to whether they require outpatient, intensive outpatient, or residential/inpatient treatment. The intensity and duration of treatment varies depending on the service provider. For example, some inpatient treatment programs, which require high resource intensity, may be only fourteen days long or can last as long as three months. The goal is often to initiate treatment and stabilize the individual. A therapeutic community program, which would be a form of residential treatment, may be low intensity but of a long duration, for example up to two years. This often involves living with other people in recovery while working or volunteering. Alternatively, a community based outpatient program can be high intensity for a short duration for patients that are reasonably stable bio-psycho-social-spiritually, or it may be low intensity and of indefinite duration for the marginalized population where continuity of care may be challenging. None of these is necessarily better or worse than the other; it all depends on where the person is at in their disease, how much support they require, what resources are available, and how closely they can adhere to the treatment recommendations.

The ASAM Criteria[3] was developed to provide guidance for treatment of Addiction and co-occurring conditions. The criteria allow clinicians and care managers to make objective decisions related to levels of care, including continuing care for Addiction, mental health, and general health care along six dimensions. They include:

> Dimension 1 – Acute Intoxication and/or Withdrawal Potential
>
> Dimension 2 – Biomedical Conditions and Complications
>
> Dimension 3 – Emotional, Behavioral, or Cognitive Conditions and Complications
>
> Dimension 4 – Readiness to Change
>
> Dimension 5 – Relapse, Continued Use, or Continued Problem Potential
>
> Dimension 6 – Recovery/Living Environment

The ASAM Criteria describe treatment as a continuum marked by levels of service from early intervention to outpatient to intensive outpatient/day patient to residential to medically managed inpatient services as follows:

> Level 0.5 Early Intervention
>
> Level 1.0 Outpatient Services and/or Agonist Maintenance (most commonly opioids)
>
> Level 2.1 Intensive Outpatient Services
>
> Level 2.5 Partial Hospitalization Services

Level 3.1 Clinically Managed Low-Intensity Residential Services

Level 3.3 Clinically Managed Population Specific High-Intensity Residential Services

Level 3.5 Clinically Managed High-Intensity Residential Services

Level 3.7 Medically Monitored Intensive In-patient Services

Level 4.0 Medically Managed Intensive In-patient Services

There is recognition in these levels of care that medical involvement in the programs themselves may be variable, especially at Levels 0.5, 2.1, 2.5, 3.1, 3.3, and 3.5. However, it is essential to appreciate that physician involvement is paramount at all levels of care. The ASAM Criteria also recognize that adolescents have different needs than adults. For example, Level 3.3 is not designated for adolescents, and instead medium-intensity with longer duration (Level 3.5) is recommended in many instances to ensure the establishment of a recovery foundation in the context of their peer group.

In each of these levels, the acuity of problems in Dimensions 1, 2, and 3 would be a determining variable. From the perspective of ongoing treatment needs, Dimensions 4, 5, and 6 are critical during the initial intervention and assessment and require close attention during continuing care, as problems in those dimensions as well would necessitate adjustment of the level of care.

It is essential for all health care providers to provide feedback when addiction-related problems are identified as an early intervention (0.5). The determination of other levels of care is directly connected to the severity of withdrawal (Dimension 1), which may or may not require medical management, and complications related to physical (Dimension 2) or mental health problems (Dimension 3).

Lack of availability of appropriate services can also bump patients into lower or higher levels of care. It is understood that for someone requiring a lower level of care, availing a higher level of care may still benefit, whereas when someone requiring a higher level of care is given a lower level of care because of financial or systemic constraints, they risk losing confidence in the treatment system. The difficulties with relapse and pessimism about treatment outcome are a direct result of a disconnection between what patients need and what they get.

Sadly, many providers and members of the public subscribe to the educational model, which implies that once you have taken a course and graduated, you should know better in the future. This model completely ignores the relapsing-remitting aspect of Addiction and is shame-based, as it inadvertently blames the person for not 'getting it' if they continue to struggle. It is also based on expectations that programs should cure which, as discussed earlier, only detracts from reality and creates resentment. It would be important for the treatment system to move away from graduation ceremonies or giving patients alumni status, as more shame is generated when there is a recurrence of the disease or relapse. It would be preferable if treatment centres encouraged continued contact and mutual support amongst those who have completed the program and provided opportunities for regular connection after the program finishes such that open dialogue of challenges continues. Similarly, the term 'aftercare', used by many providers, especially residential treatment centres, insinuates that treatment is time-limited as opposed to 'continuing care', which fits within the chronic disease model of ongoing care being necessary.

PAIN — ACUTE AND CHRONIC

Opioids are commonly prescribed for pain relief on acute and chronic bases. People with Addiction also suffer from pain and similarly require optimal treatment. Treatment of chronic pain with opioids

for non-terminal conditions when Addiction is present is controversial. No one wants their patient to suffer needlessly, but current
literature suggests that simply using escalating doses of opioids for
chronic pain often backfires.[4] In the case of pain that is unrelent-
ing, opioids ought to be a consideration as a clinical trial. Experts
recommend screening patients before starting opioids with one of
the many instruments available that often stratify risk rather than
identifying Addiction. People with Addiction requiring opioid maintenance need tighter boundaries around the amount of medication
that is dispensed to them at a time. Weekly pick-ups of long-acting
opioids are recommended in most circumstances. Short-acting medications are prescribed commonly for 'break-through' pain (acute
escalation of pain in the presence of chronic pain) at certain times,
with certain activities. It is essential to avoid short-acting medications because of rapid reinforcement being a significant factor in
increasing tolerance and worsening addiction-related problems.
Rapid reinforcement means a quick rise in the blood levels of a short-
acting opioid invariably activates the reward circuitry. It is usually
difficult, if not impossible, for a person with Addiction to recognize
when it is a pain flare-up and when it is craving. Further, people with
Addiction are well known to start taking more short-acting opioids
misguidedly in anticipation of a pain flare up.

The clinical trial of opioids, when undertaken, ought to be
directed towards proper pain relief, absence of serious side effects,
attention to the presence of aberrant behaviours, and special attention is required to the preservation or improvement of function.
Simply aiming for relief of pain is not the proper treatment for
chronic painful conditions. Further, the pain relief goal is to decrease
the pain to manageable levels rather than eliminating the pain. On
a visual analog scale, a pain score of 4-5/10 is considered reasonable
as a goal, not 0/10. If treatment is not successful in reducing pain
while maintaining function, then the clinical trial would be deemed
unsuccessful and serious consideration to discontinuing the opioids
would be essential.

Many prescribers prefer methadone or buprenorphine as the main opioid for chronic pain, though that is currently an 'off-label' indication. This means that treating chronic pain is not the officially sanctioned prescription indication for these products; however, physicians can make those decisions for individual patients in their specific circumstances. Principles of opioid maintenance therapy for opioid dependence may be followed for pain management as well. However, it must be appreciated that once a day dosing of maintenance opioids may not work for chronic pain patients and twice or three times daily administration is often needed. Adjunctive measures to reduce pain need to be a part of any treatment regimen, especially if the patient has Addiction. This includes but is not limited to physical activity (e.g., exercise, stretching, physical therapy, acupuncture, yoga and Pilates), mindfulness activities (e.g., meditation, guided relaxation, and spiritual practices), mutual support, and some form of support for the mental aspects of chronic pain (e.g., cognitive-behavioural therapy, acceptance commitment therapy, dialectical behavioural therapy).

ANTI-CRAVING MEDICATIONS

Although physicians often prescribe medications to facilitate the treatment of Addiction, there are few medications that appear to be helpful in reducing craving,[5] which is the desire to use more in the presence or absence of a substance in a person's system. Oral naltrexone, injectable naltrexone, implantable depot preparations of naltrexone, and oral acamprosate are the products currently available for addressing craving.

Naltrexone is an opioid antagonist that blocks the mu-opioid receptor, which when sitting empty is hypothesized to be a significant contributor to craving. Even though this is an opioid circuitry specific blockade, craving reduction occurs for Addiction involving various substances and behaviours in individual patients because of the commonalities in activation of the reward pathway that includes the opioid circuitry. In other words, this medication can be helpful for other manifestations of Addiction besides opioids, including for alcohol, sex, and food. For patients with Addiction involving opioids, the high affinity of naltrexone to the opioid receptor as compared to opioid agonists in general, detracts from any relief that someone may be seeking from other opioids when on naltrexone therapy. If someone does need pain management for acute injuries or surgery, the naltrexone needs to be discontinued or in emergency situations much higher doses of opioids would be required to provide relief in the presence of naltrexone.

Buprenorphine, a partial opioid agonist, appears to have benefits for decreasing craving for opioids and diminished relapse. Disulfiram, although not an anti-craving medication, has some benefit in selected cases for decreasing relapse to alcohol use. It is important to appreciate that disulfiram does not reduce craving, whereas naltrexone does. Disulfiram cannot be taken while one is still drinking, while naltrexone can be started even then. Naltrexone is effective in decreasing the volume of alcohol use even when the individual is not willing or able to abstain.

Acamprosate is hypothesized to be more useful for addressing the glutamate circuitry related problems in the brain, which are associated with mood lability and seeking drugs for relief from uncomfortable feelings. The mechanism of action is not clearly understood and the studies to establish its efficacy have been equivocal in their results. It is more useful to consider each patient individually to assess if particular circumstances for a patient are occurring, such as vulnerability to cue-induced dysphoria, which is more indicative of glutamate circuitry needing to be the target. Research continues to investigate pharmacological interventions that may help in the circuit involving corticotropin releasing factor peptide from the hypothalamus affecting the release of endorphins and ACTH from the pituitary gland.

ANTI-DEPRESSANT MEDICATIONS

Data regarding the efficacy of anti-depressants for Addiction are mixed.[6] Considerations for concurrent mood disorders or major depression include tricyclics (e.g. amitriptyline, nortriptyline, doxepin), selective serotonin reuptake inhibitors (e.g. citalopram, sertraline, fluoxetine), serotonin and norepinephrine reuptake inhibitors (e.g. duloxetine, venlafaxine), and norepinephrine-dopamine reuptake inhibitors (e.g. buproprion). Anti-depressant medications are generally not effective in the face of active Addiction and often result in undesirable side effects such as dysphoria, suicidal ideation, or uncharacteristic uncontrollable behaviour that may result in aggression or violence. The risk among adolescents and young adults while their brain is still developing has not been appreciated fully.

Depression is a common symptom of intoxication and withdrawal in people with Addiction, hence, care is required in initiating or continuing anti-depressant therapy in selected cases where there is marked functional impairment that is interfering with the individual engaging in recovery.

ANTI-ANXIETY MEDICATIONS

Selective serotonin reuptake inhibitors (SSRIs) are also thought to be helpful for anxiety and panic disorder, and are preferable to chronic use of benzodiazepines for those conditions. Buspirone, an azapirone medication, can be effective for anxiety without the abuse liability of the benzodiazepines.

It is essential to appreciate, however, that anxiety is a symptom usually related to a lot of fear. Treatment needs to be focused on identifying and dealing with the roots of fear rather than symptom suppression with anti-anxiety medications. Further, anxiety can also be a symptom of intoxication, withdrawal, and craving. Careful evaluation of individual patients is required to fully appreciate what may be happening, and all treatment approaches need to take recovery principles into consideration.

SLEEP MEDICATIONS

Medications for sleeplessness, which is a significant problem for people in the early stages of recovery, include but are not limited to sedating antidepressants (e.g. mirtazepine, amitriptyline, nortriptyline, doxepin, trazodone), atypical antipsychotics (e.g. risperidone, quetiapine, olanzepine), and over-the-counter preparations (melatonin, valerian root, Dramamine). Benzodiazepines and benzo-like sedative-hypnotics, such as zolpidem or zopiclone, have abuse liability and dependence potential; they are not recommended for treatment of insomnia for someone with Addiction. Sedating antihistamines, such as diphenhydramine or hydroxazine, and anti-nauseants, such as dimenhydrinate, can present a problem as well in exacerbating addiction-related problems due to their depressant effects on the brain and need to be avoided.

Employing healthy sleep hygiene techniques, including a set bed and waking time, darkness, a cool room, and a comfortable pillow and mattress to help sleep is an important part of recovery. Aiming for quietness and not reading or watching TV or using electronic devices in bed is also essential. Relaxing music, aroma therapy, or white noise generators can be helpful sometimes. Journal writing to process feelings and maintaining a focus on recovery will generally help normalize sleep over a few months. If insomnia is related to waking up in the middle of the night after little or restless sleep, journal writing allows thoughts and feelings to be expressed and sleep often follows.

TREATMENT PROVIDERS

The lay of the land for Addiction treatment is still diffuse and less than coherent, thus creating a lot of confusion for clients/patients and health care providers. Psychiatrists, physicians, psychologists, social workers, and counsellors continue to operate in independent silos where information about patients is not shared with other health care professionals. Moving forward, it is important to have open lines of communication between treating professionals to establish consistent care for all patients, not just those struggling with Addiction. It is also essential that health care providers use a common language of terms,[7] such as those developed by the American Society of Addiction Medicine, some of which are outlined in the Glossary.

Our discussion will now explore common psychotherapeutic approaches for Addiction, treatment modalities, and the future of health care in the context of Addiction.

Behavioural Treatment. This has been the norm in Addiction treatment for decades, although medications are sometimes added concurrently. As Addiction has been generally viewed as a behavioural disorder by social workers, psychologists and psychiatrists, it seemed to make sense to focus on behaviour modification to deal with the problems. The most common treatment approaches for Addiction have been cognitive-behavioural therapy (CBT), motivational interviewing (MI), dialectical behavioural therapy (DBT), and various forms of family therapy when it is determined that treating the individual may not be sufficient. Individual psychotherapy, regardless of specific approach, consists of a series of techniques that help people to identify their feelings and ways of thinking so they become better at coping with difficult situations.

Cognitive-behavioural therapy was developed by Dr. Aaron Beck[8] in the 1960s and has continued to evolve since then. It has become one of the most common psychotherapeutic approaches for various mental health issues, including depression, anxiety, anxiety-related disorders (e.g., obsessive-compulsive disorder, phobias, and post-traumatic stress disorder), as well as Addiction specifically related to drugs, alcohol, and eating disorders. CBT addresses the dysfunctional thought patterns that individuals carry that produce subsequent changes in feeling and behaviour. CBT works with individuals to address unrealistic thoughts by identifying them and looking at systematic ways to shift thoughts to become more rational and realistic. For example, if someone identifies that they are thinking 'I am stupid,' a cognitive-behavioural approach would be to develop reasonable alternatives to replace that thought, such as 'I am trying the best I can' or 'I am a capable person.' If thinking is more reasonable and rational, then people typically feel healthier, meaning they are less stressed, anxious, worried, or depressed, and will consequently act differently, such as more thoughtfully with less desire to escape, numb, or avoid reality.

In the context of Addiction, CBT is often used to help people identify their internal vulnerabilities for substance use, avoid these circumstances if possible, and work on other internal issues, such as depression, anxiety, or low self-esteem, which may be contributing to the desire to act out. Homework is a standard intervention within CBT that encourages the individual to take personal responsibility and accountability over their health and recovery journey. CBT is often short-term in nature, with the understanding that once individuals have learned the necessary skills and information they can continue to employ it in their lives outside of the therapeutic context. With Addiction, there is a risk that CBT can lead to an individual thinking that they can control the disease by thought blocking or substitution, when a more fundamental strategy is needed in recovery that includes surrender and acceptance.

MI was developed in 1983 by William Miller[9] and Stephen Rollnick in response to their work with problem drinkers. Motivational interviewing is a person-centred, collaborative counselling approach that seeks to focus on identifying and encouraging internal motivation for change. Rather than establishing a coercive or external motivation for change (e.g., 'Do this or else this will be the consequence'), MI works with the client to identify what they are looking for in their lives and what actions they are willing and able to take. It is the health care provider's job to draw out the client's own motivations and skills for change rather than imposing their own ideas of what 'should' happen. MI has changed over the past thirty years since its inception, and in 2009 was defined as "...a collaborative, person-centered form of guiding to elicit and strengthen motivation for change."

MI can be particularly helpful in working with Addiction because there may be a high level of denial preventing the individual from recognizing the detrimental impact substance use and/or problematic behaviours are having in their life. With MI, the health care provider works to clarify the mismatch between where clients want to be and where they are, which is where motivation comes from.

DBT is a form of psychotherapy that was originally developed by Marsha M. Linehan[10] to treat people with borderline personality disorder (BPD) and chronically suicidal individuals. DBT combines standard cognitive-behavioural techniques for emotion regulation and reality-testing with concepts of distress tolerance, acceptance, and mindful awareness largely derived from Buddhist meditative practice. It helps people focus more on the present and face the painful realities of life to develop more effective recovery strategies and practice recovery action more consistently.

With family therapy, the family, not the individual, is seen as the patient. There are still challenges in moving the focus from the identified patient (IP), or the individual with Addiction, to the family unit. The biggest challenge is that the IP typically has the most severe or disruptive problem, so the attention focuses on resolving these issues. Other family members, who are likely struggling themselves with communication, boundaries, mental health issues, conflict, self-care, or even Addiction, often do not take time or resources to focus on their own health and recovery, as discussed in Chapter 7.

Psychotherapy,[11] regardless of the specific techniques (some of which were discussed above) is a therapeutic interaction between a trained professional and a client, patient, family, couple, or group. Psychotherapy includes interactive processes between a person or group and a qualified mental health professional (psychiatrist, physician, psychologist, clinical social worker, licensed counselor, or other trained practitioner). Its purpose is the exploration of thoughts, feelings, and behaviour specifically related to identifying barriers for the purpose of problem-solving or achieving higher levels of functioning, even in the face of resistance from the client/patient. Psychotherapy aims to address the resistance by raising awareness of dissonance, to increase the individual's sense of his or her self-efficacy and well-being. Psychotherapists employ a range of techniques based on experiential relationship building, dialogue, communication, and behaviour change that are designed to improve the mental health of a client or patient, or to improve group relationships, such as in a family. Research has repeatedly shown that it is the provider-client/patient relationship based on mutual respect, trust, and unconditional positive regard that leads to healthier outcomes rather than any specific technique.

For a health care professional to be truly effective in helping the individual and family, they need to be adept at all types of psychotherapeutic strategies and be able to interchange different modes of therapy depending on the needs of the individual or family. Health care professionals that engage in active listening skills and are eclectic in their repertoire of treatment strategies will likely be more effective overall than being tied to one mode of treatment. Although the term counselling is sometimes used interchangeably with psychotherapy, it must be appreciated that counselling is generally considered to be unidirectional—information going from the provider to the client/patient—whereas psychotherapy is always bidirectional, with the therapist adjusting the approach depending on the resistance or barriers that are encountered.

Medication treatment. Another approach for the treatment of Addiction has been to use specific medications to manage significant withdrawal symptoms, during a taper plan or abstinence that is established cold turkey. As discussed in Chapter 6, withdrawal from depressants can be life-threatening and medical intervention is essential in accord with best practices established in context of current research and/or the clinical experience of the providers.

Disulfiram, a medication that makes people physically ill after the ingestion of alcohol; and methadone, a drug used for maintenance or in a taper plan for individuals coming off heroin or other opioids, are two of the older, most widely known medications used in treatment of Addiction.

Suboxone and naltrexone are other medications currently being used in Addiction treatment. Suboxone is useful to support maintenance or taper plans from opioids and naltrexone is useful for abstinence from alcohol, other drugs, and problematic behaviours. These drugs work on receptors in the brain that opioids bind to and produce their effect. As discussed previously, methadone is a pure opioid agonist and methadone maintenance treatment (MMT) is therefore sometimes called substitution therapy. Suboxone is a combination of buprenorphine, a partial agonist opioid, and naloxone, an opioid antagonist, which is only active when injected. The Suboxone formulation with naloxone, when taken as prescribed sublingually, leaves the naloxone inert, as it is not absorbed orally. However, if one tries to inject the Suboxone preparation, the naloxone interferes with the buprenorphine benefits.

Naltrexone is an opioid antagonist that can be taken orally, has a long half-life, and blocks the opioid receptor, thereby reducing craving and nullifying any agonist effects if another opioid is taken. This is why naltrexone cannot be given to someone who has to take opioids therapeutically for pain.

While medication treatment can be the preferred approach for some health care providers in working with Addiction, medications need to be used in conjunction with psychotherapy or other behavioural treatments as main interventions. Special training and licensing is required for physicians to prescribe methadone and Suboxone. It is essential to recognize that medications address only parts of the biological and psychological dimension, whereas holistic treatment requires addressing these more fully with other modalities such as nutrition, exercise, and psychotherapy, in addition to addressing the social and spiritual aspects of the disease to ensure holistic recovery.

TREATMENT MODES

Outpatient. Outpatient treatment is typically comprised of individual psychotherapy, group psychotherapy, educational programs, or a combination thereof. The term 'outpatient' refers to the fact that clients complete programming or therapy at a designated location, then return to their homes and daily life, they do not live in a facility. No significant time off work is required for outpatient treatment, although in the early days of recovery this is something health care professionals can consider recommending to give individuals an opportunity to connect with their recovery. Much like someone who has been diagnosed with cancer or another long-term condition, it may be beneficial to have time away from work to focus on treatment and develop a recovery routine. The recommended period for an initial leave of absence is a minimum of three months with Addiction, as this is the minimum required for cravings to subside, recovery activities to become more habitual, and for the brain to begin to develop alternate pathways.

Outpatient programs can be extremely beneficial as an opportunity to learn about Addiction as a primary, chronic brain disease; a place to start exploring feelings and challenges more honestly; and are a place where health care providers can provide recommendations and feedback on the role of the disease in one's life and the holistic recovery options available. The biggest advantage of outpatient treatment is that recovery is established in the individual's home community, which is necessary over the longer term of an individual's lifetime even if more intensive, residential treatment services may have been required at some point.

The drawback to outpatient programs is that they may not be enough support, particularly if someone is struggling to maintain abstinence from substance(s) and problem behaviours. Often clients will insist on starting with outpatient programming, perhaps because it is often viewed as easier. This is because there is less accountability and may often be chosen by individuals in the pre-contemplative or contemplative stages of change, when they have little to no appreciation of the problem Addiction is in their life and do not want to spend a lot of time or resources on treatment. However, some individuals who have limited time to be away from work, financial limitations, or family restrictions will choose outpatient programming and their level of motivation and desire for change is high. In all of these cases, it is recommended to start with outpatient programming with the caveat that if struggles continue at the same level or worsen over the next three months, a more intensive treatment approach must be considered.

Intensive Outpatient Programs (IOP). Adding the word 'intensive' to outpatient programming brings a new level of accountability, time commitment, and dedication to recovery action. While IOPs vary in terms of length, content, and structure, often they are full-time day or daily evening programs run several times a week for a period of weeks or months. IOPs often involve a combination of education, group therapy, and individual therapy covering topics such as the impact of substance on the brain and body, relapse prevention, dealing with emotions and stress, and family issues such as communication and boundaries. Individuals still go home at the end of the day during an IOP and are thus responsible for daily living needs and continuing care outside of the context of the program. However, there is a greater level of structure and time in an IOP and often they are scheduled so that individuals need to take time off work or school to participate, but the duration is shorter than that required for attending residential programs. IOPs are often used for individuals who are struggling with outpatient programming or for those who have been to residential treatment and continue to face challenges that are difficult for them to cope with.

As a health care provider, it is important to be aware of what treatment patients have attended in the past and do an assessment of where they are currently at in their recovery to make an appropriate treatment recommendation. Considering their stage and readiness of change; previous treatment; current challenges; financial and time limitations; and the client's preference for treatment are important in determining what the recommendation may be, especially in the context of what may be available and feasible. Resources for treatment remain limited and costs continue to be a huge barrier as insurance plans—public or private—are not appreciative of what quality treatment programs may be needed.

Residential treatment. This is the most prudent option for clients/patients who are open to going away to a live-in treatment facility for a period. Often by this point people have tried outpatient, intensive outpatient, or a combination and are continuing to struggle with daily living and substance use/problem behaviours. Residential treatment is essential for those who have an unstable social environment and for those who are in the severe stages of progression of their disease. Those that may need a medically supervised withdrawal management, arrangements for residential treatment immediately following the detoxification would be the most prudent course of action. Residential treatment facilities often have psychologists, social workers, nurses, and counsellors on-site, with variable levels of physician and psychiatrist consultations that are done routinely or electively in certain situations. The patient lives there full-time for anywhere from twenty-one days to twelve months. Programming is typically a combination of education, skills training, individual therapy, group therapy, recreational activities, chores, and 12-step meetings. Meals and lodging are provided and there is limited contact with the outside world for the duration of the stay. Most residential treatment facilities include a family component to their program, where family members come to engage in treatment and programming.

Residential treatment facilities are not created equal and come in a variety of models, lengths of stay, cost, and approaches, especially in relation to the training and qualifications of their staff. Thus, it is important for health care providers to have knowledge of the available options for patients, which may come from visits to the facility or with the core clinical staff to become familiar with their treatment methods. It is also important for patients to do some research into the available options and discuss the potential benefits and drawbacks with their health care provider(s) before making a decision.

It is essential that neither the health care provider nor patient view residential treatment as the 'cure-all' or 'fix' for Addiction. As we have discussed in depth, Addiction is a disease of the brain that cannot be cured, but healthy recovery is possible with continued effort and action. The risk of viewing residential treatment as the treatment and cure is that continuing recovery action will stop or dramatically diminish upon returning home, which makes relapse more likely. For those who believe residential treatment is a cure, there can be a lot of shame and self-blame that occurs in the context of relapse, plus a lot of blaming of the treatment facility or program, which can lead some to say that residential treatment does not work. Residential treatment needs to be viewed for what it is: a stepping-stone and opportunity to establish a foundation of recovery. After completion of the program, a strong continuing care plan consisting of individual therapy, group therapy, community support meetings, and holistic recovery action must be in place to continue building on this foundation, especially in the context of vigilance regarding relapse-warning signs that can be addressed, thus ensuring relapse-prevention.

Mandated treatment. As willingness is a key to accepting the diagnosis of Addiction and engagement in the treatment and recovery process, people often question the validity of mandated treatment.[12] However, it has been demonstrated repeatedly to be beneficial. Individuals who are mandated for treatment typically have as good or better treatment outcomes, higher attendance rates, and remain in treatment for longer periods. During mandated treatment, a sense of willingness to look at one's self and surrender often develops as people have a chance to detoxify and have a period of abstinence from substance, and time to focus on one's self with no distractions. People have the opportunity to face the unmanageability of their lives and develop a relationship with themselves and their higher power that, for some, can continue once their mandated treatment period has ceded. For those who never have the opportunity of mandated treatment, how, when, or if this time of detoxification and self-reflection arises will vary.

The important point is that willingness cannot be forced, coaxed, or threatened into existence. Rather, it must develop organically within the person struggling with Addiction, within the context of accountability. Professional licensing bodies and employers can often exert a pressure in the context of accountability, which ultimately helps individuals get into and maintain recovery. Concerned family members and health care professionals who sign themselves up for the mission of rescuing the struggling person with Addiction create more damage in the process as they push their loved one or patient deeper into the shame they are currently residing in. The process of recovery will begin when it needs to and unfold how it needs to using the framework of holistic recovery.

BARRIERS TO TREATMENT

Funding Limitations. Worldwide, there is a lack of financial support from governments for Addiction and mental health treatment. For those who have insurance, coverage is often sparse and not sufficient for funding residential treatment, intensive outpatient programs, or even certain avenues of outpatient programming. Government funded programs for Addiction are often short-term and behavioural focused, not allowing for an exploration of Addiction beyond substance and to look at bio-psycho-social-spiritual elements of recovery and treatment. While trying to provide resources, often such programs reinforce the 'bad behaviour and poor choices' approach to Addiction, which only serves to increase shame and self-blame, and reinforce disease activity. All too often, those who are most willing and in need of assistance do not have the financial resources to support treatment, so they are caught in a perpetual cycle of disease.

Advocacy at the local, provincial/state, and federal level is the way for health care providers and patients to promote change to a stale system. Writing letters to representatives, attending conferences or meetings where health care providers and funders are present, and advocating for a holistic approach to treatment will hopefully shift the tide to appreciating Addiction as a primary, chronic brain disease. This in turn will create more open and honest dialogues about the role of Addiction in society, without stigma or judgment.

Even though Canadians are used to health care being covered under provincial health insurance plans, public funding for Addiction and mental health is generally sub-optimal and the staff training and manpower resources are limited in public facilities and create a lot of demoralization among patients accessing those programs. This can mean a lot of turnaround in providers which disrupts the patient's sense of safety and trust. Often people have to incur many out-of-pocket expenses to get quality care. The problems have been even worse in the United States, which led to the development and promulgation of the Mental Health Parity and Addiction Treatment Equity Act by Congress under the guidance of Patrick Kennedy. However, challenges remain in implementation, and managed care barriers exist in trying to get approvals from insurers for treatment for Addiction and mental health problems.

Lack of Training. All health care providers, whether they are medical doctors, social workers, or psychologists, receive little to no training in assessing and treating Addiction during their educational degree programs. Most education in this area comes on the job and, as we have seen, approaches are diverse and inconsistent. Many are taught from old knowledge and information that has since been proven non-factual or ineffective.

For health care providers to be on the same page, courses on Addiction Medicine, that emphasize proper assessment and treatment need to be provided at a school and training level, so health care providers entering their respective fields are approaching this disease in a consistent manner. Patients become confused as they bounce between health care providers to try to find treatment, yet receive contradictory information at every turn. More students are turning to specialized Addiction training programs or seeking out practicums in agencies or with health care providers who focus on Addiction to gain knowledge in this area, recognizing that it is a major part of what they will encounter in real-world practice. Training programs for physicians are being developed with oversight and accreditation by the American Board of Addiction Medicine (ABAM) and ASAM continues to be the leading organization in North America to provide state-of-the-art training. In Canada, efforts are being made by the Canadian Centre on Substance Abuse (CCSA) in Ottawa and the Centre for Addiction and Mental Health (CAMH) in Toronto, however, there is a long ways to go. A grassroots initiative, Foundation for Addiction and Mental Health (FAMH), has also been established in Calgary.

Silo Practices. Once health care providers are in their fields and practicing, many do so independently and have little or no contact with other health care providers. Clinical consultation, feedback from others, and having as much information about clients and patients as possible are all reasons that consultation and discussion are important. More agencies that have many health care providers from different professions on-site and working together are popping up, but have certainly yet to become the norm. In the meantime, taking initiative to affiliate with other health care providers, get signed consent/releases from clients/patients to consult and collaborate with other medical professionals, and joining professional groups where clinical discussions and professional dialogue can be beneficial. Ideally, an integrated team approach works best, which was the impetus behind our developing the HUM program.

THE HEALTH CARE PROVIDER'S
OWN HEALTH AND RECOVERY

No gene pool is uncontaminated from the risk for Addiction.[13] This also means that no professional population, including health care providers, is immune to the risks. There are health care providers working in the Addiction field who are struggling from Addiction themselves. Some are aware of this, in recovery, and come to the field in the context of their own personal growth and development. Others are unaware, not in recovery, and continue to work with those struggling with Addiction, with equivocal results, as their own struggles sadly interfere with their ability to provide optimum care.

The risk for abuse or unhealthy use (hazardous or harmful) of prescription medications is higher for health care professionals, due to their availability and ease of access, so having an untreated Addiction problem while working in the health care field, even outside of Addiction, becomes problematic. It is essential that health care providers be aware of their vulnerabilities and have a health and wellness plan in place to deal with any issues that arise. Health care providers, to perform their duties effectively, may put on a professional mask that supposedly shelters any personal issues from affecting their work. However, the risk is that this mask is never taken off and the façade of being okay and healthy continues once the workday is done, even though personal challenges and struggles may exist. Holistic recovery is not just applicable to Addiction and mental health issues, but is important for everyone, including health care providers, to engage in recovery to prevent burnout and vulnerabilities from manifesting into bigger issues. Burnout is sometimes also called compassion fatigue. It is essential that providers seek proper assessment and treatment when facing difficulties, especially related to Addiction and mental health issues, rather than making a geographical move or just time off for stress, which may or may not address reality.

Programs for professionals needing assessment, treatment and monitoring are available in many jurisdictions through regulatory bodies or professional associations.[14] Many programs recognize the chronic nature of the disease of Addiction, so monitoring is done for at least five years and is extended for those wanting to continue or having difficulty. Accountability is an essential component of recovery and urine drug monitoring is included in these programs, with appropriate clinical care that includes individual and group psychotherapy, together with mutual support programs.

HEALTH CARE PROVIDERS EDUCATION AND TRAINING

Despite the persistent, known challenges that exist and persist among patients, education and training of physicians, nurses, psychologists, social workers, and other counselors remains deficient in relation to addiction-related and mental health problems. Even the bio-psycho-social-spiritual model of care can emphasize one over the others, whereas each aspect needs to be given as much weight and consideration. As much as different professional groups and university faculties offer courses leading to degrees, added qualifications, or certification, some of the teaching on Addiction can reinforce biases that are not necessarily in the best interest of the clients or patients coming for care. It also results in a lot of confusion such that policy makers and the public are left thinking that they have to choose between competing philosophies and models. The challenge remains for all professional training programs to provide more holistic training and promote the provision of holistic care in an integrated team environment. The patients need consistent and congruent feedback and direction to approach recovery from Addiction and mental health problems in a healthy, balanced manner without shame or fear being the motivating factors for change in thinking, feelings, and behaviours.

For physicians in North America, the American Board of Addiction Medicine (ABAM)[15] is providing leadership and direction in training and certification of physicians for the ultimate benefit to individuals, families, and society as a whole. The Certificant of the Canadian Society of Addiction Medicine (CCSAM) designation accepts the ABAM examination as its base qualification, as well as the examination developed and delivered by the International Society of Addiction Medicine (ISAM) that provides the CISAM designation.[16] The Diplomate of ABAM (DABAM) designation is expected to be recognized by the American Board of Medical Specialties in the near future.

THE FUTURE OF ADDICTION CARE: INDIVIDUALIZED TREATMENT PLANS

As our knowledge and understanding of Addiction grows, it is increasingly necessary that patients and health care providers appreciate that treatment for Addiction needs to be tailored to the individual and their needs. It is also important to add that this individualized treatment plan needs to occur in the context of abstinence from all mood-altering substances in the context of holistic recovery. One can stop looking for the best treatment for everyone and focus on what is the best treatment for the individual in their current context, keeping an open mind such that treatment can be adjusted and modified to suit one's needs over time.

All of the psychotherapeutic approaches described above, as well as ones that have not been mentioned (e.g., humanistic therapy, solution-focused therapy, existential therapy, gestalt therapy to name a few), have a potential role to play in Addiction treatment but cannot be used in isolation or without consideration of the needs and stage of change of the patient. In the early days of recovery, a focus on medical stabilization may be the number one priority, so some behavioural interventions, combined with pharmacotherapy options, may be employed. As the individual stabilizes, an eclectic blend of many treatment approaches would be utilized to explore the biological, psychological, emotional, social, and spiritual realms of recovery.

The attention of physicians in all parts of the world to issues involving pathological use of reward-inducing substances has historically been skewed toward the medical/surgical complications of substance use (e.g., liver and esophageal damage from drinking alcohol, lung damage from smoking drugs, infections such as HIV, hepatitis, and others). It needs instead to focus on the underlying illness (Addiction), in which individuals have a pathological relationship with a source of reward or relief because of how their brain operates differently from other persons who do not have Addiction. The rewards and relief for people with Addiction comes from indiscriminate excess or obsessive restriction and control, which may be hard for others to understand who may view that as bad or stupid behaviour.

Treatment by physicians and other health care providers needs to focus on what makes the user unique, not the fact that they are using, since high frequency and high volume exposure to rewards happens for many people who do not have Addiction (e.g., heavy drinkers, gamblers, or overeaters). They may have significant health consequences because of their behaviour but do not have a brain disease that involves preoccupation, craving, enhanced cue response, and selective preference of particular behaviours to the exclusion of others. The treatment needs to be individualized so that those who do not have Addiction are given education to assist in changing their hazardous or harmful using, whereas those with Addiction need to be educated and provided professional treatment with individual and group psychotherapy in a continuing care framework that includes mutual peer support. In this context, slips and relapses would be processed as the disease becoming active and requiring more intervention, rather than blaming oneself or the individual for behaving badly. Pharmacotherapy options also need to be considered in individual context rather than polarized advocacy for agonist maintenance treatment or always insisting on complete abstinence. Abstinence itself can be followed as 'pursuit of restraint' with incremental improvement with awareness rather than not recommending it at all or penalizing an individual for faltering.

Individual, group, family, and experiential therapies, such as art/music/movement therapy and occupational therapy, and complementary/integrative medicine approaches including meditation, relaxation training, yoga, acupuncture, all have merit in the treatment of Addiction. As we learn more about Addiction as a brain disease, there needs to be more attention placed on offering pharmacotherapy options to patients to address some of the underlying neurobiological aberrations in the brains of persons with addiction associated with alcohol or other substances. These pharmacotherapies need to be integrated with psycho-social-spiritual approaches and must be understood as also affecting the underlying biology.

Hence, a flexible and individualized treatment plan can be put into effect using each method when it is most efficacious, as opposed to an either-or approach. Performance measures for physicians and other health care providers who work with individuals with Addiction need to look at holistic recovery approaches rather than blindly following protocols for substance-specific issues. More effective pharmacotherapies that address the addictive process itself are needed to maximize the patient's chances at long-lasting success, including impaired control, heightened cue reactivity, and helping to employ healthier decisional balance, or directly address the actions of ethanol on reward circuitry.

Treatment may consist of residential, partial hospitalization, intensive outpatient, and general outpatient approaches for persons diagnosed with drug dependence (Addiction) and behavioural aspects of Addiction, such as food, sex, and relationships, must be addressed in all treatment programs.

Harm reduction, which is a focus on reducing the addiction-related harms or adverse consequences of the disease, can be woven into service delivery even while the individual is in the pre-contemplation or contemplation stage of change for overall recovery. This can be done even though motivation for abstinence may or may not be evident beyond addressing specific substance-related issues. The ASAM definition of harm reduction is in the glossary.

One of the most fundamental implications of treating Addiction as a brain disease is that treatment approaches must resemble those for general medical care. Since Addiction is primary, chronic disease involving brain functioning, it is appropriate for physicians to be intimately involved in its diagnosis and treatment. Models of care in Western medicine are for a person with a physical or psychological complaint to present it to a physician, who, licensed to practice medicine and surgery, either prescribes a medication or proposes a surgical remedy. The highest quality medical care for all chronic diseases, including diabetes, heart diseases, and cancer, includes medical pharmacological, emotional, and cognitive interventions. Of course, many brain diseases that involve emotion, cognition, or interpersonal relations and affect psychosocial functioning even if specific physiological dysfunction cannot be identified, are treated with psychiatric methods including individual, family, or group psychotherapy, one or another modality of talk therapy, in addition to or instead of medication management.

The *Performance Measures for the Treatment of Substance Use Disorders* developed by the Physician Consortium on Practice Improvement of the American Medical Association[17] outlines that in cases of diagnosed alcohol dependence and opioid dependence, physicians should document that they have discussed with patients the option for both counselling interventions and medication management to address their health problem. Pharmacotherapies have been developed and approved for clinical use by the US Food and Drug Administration for the treatment of Addiction involving alcohol, nicotine, and opioids. Medications are under development for the treatment of Addiction involving cannabinoids and stimulants. There have been clear parallels identified in neurochemistry, neurophysiology, and neuroimaging research between Addiction associated with stimulants and Addiction associated with gambling. Many think that when an effective and safe medication is identified to treat stimulant dependence, it will prove effective in the treatment of Addiction involving gambling.

Advances are being made in genetic testing that may allow us to better understand what pharmacotherapeutic approaches may be most beneficial to which patients rather than using medications as a trial and error as it is the current norm, with limitations in understanding of mechanisms of action and individual variability.

As Addiction is a brain disease involving reward, motivation, memory, and related brain circuitry, it is reasonable to expect that the future will see broader use of a wider range of pharmacotherapy options targeting that circuitry. New medications will be discovered, as has been the case in medicine for the past fifty years, and biomedical science will drive an improvement in treatment outcomes and population health by providing clinicians with broader options for treatment of addiction. Licensed independent practitioners with prescribing authority will be more comfortable with prescribing therapeutic agents for a patient's Addiction. There will be more medical options for management of this illness, more medical professionals engaged with the treatment of this illness, and more adoption of the pharmacological therapies. Their use will be appropriately integrated with psychosocial interventions including talk therapies, which result from expanded pharmaceutical research into improved paths to recovery.

Many of the changes in the basic approach to Addiction require viewing it as a medical and public health problem more so than a social, criminological, or public safety problem. Associated changes in health care training to address this significant chronic illness continue to be discussed broadly in policy circles. Trends toward medicalization of Addiction will involve it being treated in ways more akin to other medical conditions by the same professionals and in settings where other medical professionals work and where patients go to see them. It will also use the same mechanisms of payment for services that are used when patients receive professional help for other medical conditions.

Considering Addiction as a single condition involving impairment in behavioural control means that what is wrong with the person is not what they are doing, or what they could do, but how their brain responds to exposure to substances or activities that activate their reward, motivation, memory, and related circuitry. Most specifically, it is what happens in interactions among reward, motivation, memory, and other circuitry, resulting in impulsive or compulsive engagement in substance use and other activities. Impaired control over such behaviours due to enhanced drive and impairments in the ability to inhibit intense drives aggravate Addiction. The intense compulsion in the context of a cued conditioned response to engage in a given pursuit of reward or relief perpetuates the disease. For a person with Addiction, the pursuit of reward is not only driven by the availability of the substance or other behaviours that can produce a rewarding brain response, but also by a pathological intensity of memories of experiences with the source of reward. This is coupled with apparent amnesia or minimization of negative consequences, a profound response to cues associated with reward, and a profound focusing of behaviours on those associated with seeking, finding, and using a specific behaviour to stimulate brain reward circuitry to the exclusion of other behavioural options that could be available to the individual. Behaviour becomes all about drinking, using drugs, gambling, eating, purging, or exercising, because the salience of the behaviour to pursue such sources of reward, or relief, is intensified by complex patterns of brain activity. Any potential tempering of that incentive salience from frontal lobe areas that convey judgment, planning, foresight, delay of gratification, and impulse control is diminished in cases of addiction, especially in adolescents and young adults who do not have fully developed frontal lobe circuitry.

A clinical approach that views Addiction as Addiction understands that individuals with this disease can and do switch from one unhealthy source of reward or relief to another. When Addiction is understood as a unitary condition and not a collection of 'addictions' then the concept of switching addictions takes on a different hue: it is Addiction that the affected person has, and the switch is among the many manifestations of reward or relief offered to the patient by different substances or behaviours, not among various separate health conditions.

CHAPTER SUMMARY

The recognition that Addiction is a primary, chronic disease that has broad manifestations requires that assessment be comprehensive and continue on an ongoing basis in a therapeutic environment. As the disease has been recognized to express itself along biological, psychological, social, and spiritual dimensions, assessment and treatment need to be designed with these in mind. A comprehensive assessment and individualized continuing care treatment approach allows tailoring the treatment to individual needs within a chronic disease framework.

Common psychotherapeutic approaches for Addiction treatment were explored in this chapter as well as various treatment modalities depending on the needs of the individual and available resources. Ultimately, a unified approach to Addiction treatment in a chronic disease framework of ongoing, continuing care needs to be the common standard of care. In this treatment approach, the emphasis is on tailoring treatment to the individual and recognizing that Addiction is Addiction—a unitary disease with multiple manifestations and associated with any of a number of pathological sources of reward and relief.

This chapter also provided information about the ASAM criteria, a framework and text that was developed to provide guidance for treatment of Addiction and other substance-related and co-occurring conditions. They allow clinicians and care managers to make objective decisions related to levels of care, including continuing care for addiction, mental health, and general health care. These criteria describe treatment as a continuum marked by levels of service from early intervention to outpatient, to intensive outpatient/day patient, to residential, to medically managed inpatient services. Barriers to treatment were addressed and a vision for the future of Addiction care with individualized treatment plans was explored.

Chapter 9: Summary and Conclusions

Our hope is that this book provides you greater understanding of Addiction as a primary, chronic brain disease. With appropriate assessment and treatment, there is hope for a better quality of life, more so than with other chronic diseases. Addiction is about differences in the brain functioning of people with the disease, not about their specific behaviours. To treat Addiction adequately, it is critical to understand the brain, as it is involved with everything people do including how they think, feel, behave, and interact. It must also be recognized that Addiction is not just a brain disease. Beyond the biological aspect, the disease manifestations occur along psychological, social, and spiritual dimensions, and therefore optimal treatment is holistic in each of these areas.

The definition of Addiction (found in Appendix A) was approved in 2011 by ASAM and is based on extensive review of current scientific work as well as lessons learned by experienced clinicians and experts from research and clinical practice and was used as a framework in this book. Included is an in-depth look at the characteristics of Addiction, which include the inability to consistently abstain, impairment in behavioural control, craving, diminished recognition of significant problems with one's behaviours and interpersonal relationships, and a dysfunctional emotional response. Like other chronic diseases, Addiction often involves cycles of relapse and remission. Without treatment or engagement in recovery activities, Addiction is progressive and can result in disability or premature death.

THE COSTS OF ADDICTION

Addiction and mental health problems continue to exact a heavy toll from individuals, families, and society as a whole. With the advent of the internet and smart phones, availability of various forms of reward and relief are instantly at people's fingertips. It is important to start an ongoing dialogue and ask: What is healthy? Where are the risks? It was proposed by Anne Wilson Schaef[1] many years ago that our "aliveness" as human beings is in jeopardy in the context of an "addictive system" that is performance driven towards growth and having more, without recognizing clearly what the consequences are. As is said, 'the road to hell is often paved with good intentions.'

National and international institutions are tabulating the societal costs of problems related to Addiction and mental health, however, there is no way to put a price on the mental anguish that individuals, families, and communities live with every day. Action happens only when people realize that someone else's personal costs are also our own as members of society, and that people have to move forward collectively.

THE PROMISES OF RECOVERY

'I want it, but it just seems like so much work' are the words health care providers hear time and again when recovery concepts are discussed with patients. Even health care providers sometimes throw up their hands and say that this problem is too difficult to address. Sadly, this is when the opportunities for change are missed because, external barriers notwithstanding, often the barriers are within the providers themselves. As health care providers, it is important to look at our own issues and motivations for what is done in practice, which can then translate into a more empathetic, understanding, accepting, patient-centred approach to health care. Dr. Gordon Bell (1911-2005) provided exemplary leadership in a hostile environment[2] to open the Donwood Institute, which was North America's first public hospital for the treatment of Addiction involving alcohol and drugs.

Addiction professionals and persons in recovery know the hope that is found in recovery. For the struggling person with Addiction, the promises of recovery seem amorphous and unattainable. Thoughts of a lifestyle outside of active Addiction produce fear, anxiety, and shame. However, once one begins to put some trust and faith in the recovery process, a new world opens up that was previously unimaginable. As an example, the Foundation for Addiction and Mental Health[3] (FAMH) in Calgary, Alberta, is slowly developing a grassroots movement to address stigma, provide education, build networks, and promote understanding and have appreciation of the Addiction is Addiction framework together with problems related to mental health and chronic pain.

Over time, relationships grow and transform; people feel connected, serene, and peaceful; matters they once obsessed about quiet in the mind; fear lessens; cravings for relief or reward seeking subside; intuition guides situations that were once baffling; trust and faith in a higher power develops; and life opens up a new realm of possibility and opportunity. These are the promises of recovery.

The concept of recovery can be simplified to healthy lifestyle principles for all aspects of one's being, to live with honesty, humility, acceptance, clear boundaries, and caring action with compassion towards oneself and others. Peace, harmony, and contentment are natural by-products of a balanced life on its own terms.

Appendix A: Long Definition of Addiction from the American Society of Addiction Medicine

Addiction is a primary, chronic disease of brain reward, motivation, memory, and related circuitry. Addiction affects neurotransmission and interactions within reward structures of the brain, including the nucleus accumbens, anterior cingulate cortex, basal forebrain and amygdala, such that motivational hierarchies are altered and addictive behaviors, which may or may not include alcohol and other drug use, supplant healthy, self-care related behaviors. Addiction also affects neurotransmission and interactions between cortical and hippocampal circuits and brain reward structures, such that the memory of previous exposures to rewards (such as food, sex, alcohol and other drugs) leads to a biological and behavioral response to external cues, in turn triggering craving and/or engagement in addictive behaviors.

The neurobiology of addiction encompasses more than the neurochemistry of reward. The frontal cortex of the brain and underlying white matter connections between the frontal cortex and circuits of reward, motivation and memory are fundamental in the manifestations of altered impulse control, altered judgment, and the dysfunctional pursuit of rewards (which is often experienced by the affected person as a desire to "be normal") seen in addiction—despite cumulative adverse consequences experienced from engagement in substance use and other addictive behaviors. The frontal lobes are important in inhibiting impulsivity and in assisting individuals to appropriately delay gratification. When persons with addiction manifest problems in deferring gratification, there is a neurological locus of these problems in the frontal cortex. Frontal lobe morphology, connectivity, and functioning are still in the process of maturation during adolescence and young adulthood, and early exposure to substance use is another significant factor in the development of addiction. Many neuroscientists believe that developmental morphology is the basis that makes early-life exposure to substances such an important factor.

Genetic factors account for about half of the likelihood that an individual will develop addiction. Environmental factors interact with the person's biology and affect the extent to which genetic factors exert their influence. Resiliencies the individual acquires (through parenting or later life experiences) can affect the extent to which genetic predispositions lead to the behavioral and other manifestations of addiction. Culture also plays a role in how addiction becomes actualized in persons with biological vulnerabilities to the development of addiction.

Other factors that can contribute to the appearance of addiction, leading to its characteristic bio-psycho-socio-spiritual manifestations, include:

a. The presence of an underlying biological deficit in the function of reward circuits, such that drugs and behaviors which enhance reward function are preferred and sought as reinforcers;

b. The repeated engagement in drug use or other addictive behaviors, causing neuroadaptation in motivational circuitry leading to impaired control over further drug use or engagement in addictive behaviors;

c. Cognitive and affective distortions, which impair perceptions and compromise the ability to deal with feelings, resulting in significant self-deception;

d. Disruption of healthy social supports and problems in interpersonal relationships which impact the development or impact of resiliencies;

e. Exposure to trauma or stressors that overwhelm an individual's coping abilities;

f. Distortion in meaning, purpose and values that guide attitudes, thinking and behavior;

g. Distortions in a person's connection with self, with others and with the transcendent (referred to as God by many, the Higher Power by 12-steps groups, or higher consciousness by others); and

h. The presence of co-occurring psychiatric disorders in persons who engage in substance use or other addictive behaviors.

Addiction is characterized by:

a. **Inability to consistently Abstain**;

b. **Impairment in Behavioral control**;

c. **Craving**; or increased "hunger" for drugs or rewarding experiences;

d. **Diminished recognition of significant problems** with one's behaviors and interpersonal relationships; and

e. **A dysfunctional Emotional response**.

The **power of external cues** to trigger craving and drug use, as well as to increase the frequency of engagement in other potentially addictive behaviors, is also a characteristic of addiction, with the hippocampus being important in memory of previous euphoric or dysphoric experiences, and with the amygdala being important in having motivation concentrate on selecting behaviors associated with these past experiences.

Although some believe that the difference between those who have addiction, and those who do not, is the *quantity* or *frequency* of alcohol/drug use, engagement in addictive behaviors (such as gambling or spending), or exposure to other external rewards (such as food or sex), a characteristic aspect of addiction is the *qualitative way* in which the individual responds to such exposures, stressors and environmental cues. A particularly pathological aspect of *the way* that persons with addiction pursue substance use or external rewards is that preoccupation with, obsession with and/or pursuit of rewards (e.g., alcohol and other drug use) persist despite the accumulation of adverse consequences. These manifestations can occur compulsively or impulsively, as a reflection of impaired control.

Persistent risk and/or recurrence of relapse, after periods of abstinence, is another fundamental feature of addiction. This can be triggered by exposure to rewarding substances and behaviors, by exposure to environmental cues to use, and by exposure to emotional stressors that trigger heightened activity in brain stress circuits.

In addiction there is a significant impairment in executive functioning, which manifests in problems with perception, learning, impulse control, compulsivity, and judgment. People with addiction often manifest a lower readiness to change their dysfunctional behaviors despite mounting concerns expressed by significant others in their lives; and display an apparent lack of appreciation of the magnitude of cumulative problems and complications. The still developing frontal lobes of adolescents may both compound these deficits in executive functioning and predispose youngsters to engage in "high risk" behaviors, including engaging in alcohol or other drug use. The profound drive or craving to use substances or engage in apparently rewarding behaviors, which is seen in many patients with addiction, underscores the compulsive or avolitional aspect of this disease. This is the connection with "powerlessness" over addiction and "unmanageability" of life, as is described in Step 1 of 12-steps programs.

Addiction is more than a behavioral disorder. Features of addiction include aspects of a person's behaviors, cognitions, emotions, and interactions with others, including a person's ability to relate to members of their family, to members of their community, to their own psychological state, and to things that transcend their daily experience.

Behavioral manifestations and complications of addiction, primarily due to impaired control, can include:

a. Excessive use and/or engagement in addictive behaviors, at higher frequencies and/or quantities than the person intended, often associated with a persistent desire for and unsuccessful attempts at behavioral control;

b. Excessive time lost in substance use or recovering from the effects of substance use and/or engagement in addictive behaviors, with significant adverse impact on social and occupational functioning (e.g. the development of interpersonal relationship problems or the neglect of responsibilities at home, school or work);

c. Continued use and/or engagement in addictive behaviors, despite the presence of persistent or recurrent physical or psychological problems which may have been caused or exacerbated by substance use and/or related addictive behaviors;

d. A narrowing of the behavioral repertoire focusing on rewards that are part of addiction; and

e. An apparent lack of ability and/or readiness to take consistent, ameliorative action despite recognition of problems.

Cognitive changes in addiction can include:

a. Preoccupation with substance use;

b. Altered evaluations of the relative benefits and detriments associated with drugs or rewarding behaviors; and

c. The inaccurate belief that problems experienced in one's life are attributable to other causes rather than being a predictable consequence of addiction.

Emotional changes in addiction can include:

a. Increased anxiety, dysphoria and emotional pain;

b. Increased sensitivity to stressors associated with the recruitment of brain stress systems, such that "things seem more stressful" as a result; and

c. Difficulty in identifying feelings, distinguishing between feelings and the bodily sensations of emotional arousal, and describing feelings to other people (sometimes referred to as alexithymia).

The emotional aspects of addiction are quite complex. Some persons use alcohol or other drugs or pathologically pursue other rewards because they are seeking "positive reinforcement" or the creation of a positive emotional state ("euphoria"). Others pursue substance use or other rewards because they have experienced relief from negative emotional states ("dysphoria"), which constitutes "negative reinforcement." Beyond the initial experiences of reward and relief, there is a **dysfunctional emotional state** present in most cases of addiction that is associated with the persistence of engagement with addictive behaviors. The state of addiction is not the same as the state of intoxication. When anyone experiences mild intoxication through the use of alcohol or other drugs, or when one engages non-pathologically in potentially addictive behaviors such as gambling or eating, one may experience a "high", felt as a "positive" emotional state associated with increased dopamine and opioid peptide activity in reward circuits. After such an experience, there is a neurochemical rebound, in which the reward function does not simply revert to baseline, but often drops below the original levels. This is usually not consciously perceptible by the individual and is not necessarily associated with functional impairments.

Over time, repeated experiences with substance use or addictive behaviors are not associated with ever-increasing reward circuit activity and are not as subjectively rewarding. Once a person experiences withdrawal from drug use or comparable behaviors, there is an anxious, agitated, dysphoric, and labile emotional experience, related to suboptimal reward and the recruitment of brain and hormonal stress systems, which is associated with withdrawal from virtually all pharmacological classes of addictive drugs. While tolerance develops to the "high", tolerance does not develop to the emotional "low" associated with the cycle of intoxication and withdrawal. Thus, in addiction, persons repeatedly attempt to create a "high"—but what they mostly experience is a deeper and deeper "low." While anyone may "want" to get "high", those with addiction feel a "need" to use the addictive substance or engage in the addictive behavior in order to try to resolve their dysphoric emotional state or their physiological symptoms of withdrawal. Persons with addiction compulsively use even though it may not make them feel good, in some cases long after the pursuit of "rewards" is not actually pleasurable.[5] Although people from any culture may choose to "get high" from one or another activity, it is important to appreciate that addiction is not solely a function of choice. Simply put, addiction is not a desired condition.

As addiction is a chronic disease, periods of relapse, which may interrupt spans of remission, are a common feature of addiction. It is also important to recognize that return to drug use or pathological pursuit of rewards is not inevitable.

Clinical interventions can be quite effective in altering the course of addiction. Close monitoring of the behaviors of the individual and contingency management, sometimes including behavioral consequences for relapse behaviors, can contribute to positive clinical outcomes. Engagement in health promotion activities which promote personal responsibility and accountability, connection with others, and personal growth also contribute to recovery. It is important to recognize that **addiction can cause disability or premature death, especially when left untreated or treated inadequately**.

The qualitative ways in which the brain and behavior respond to drug exposure and engagement in addictive behaviors are different at later stages of addiction than in earlier stages, indicating progression, which may not be overtly apparent. As is the case with other chronic diseases, the condition must be monitored and managed over time to:

a. Decrease the frequency and intensity of relapses;

b. Sustain periods of remission; and

c. Optimize the person's level of functioning during periods of remission.

In some cases of addiction, medication management can improve treatment outcomes. In most cases of addiction, the integration of psychosocial rehabilitation and ongoing care with evidence-based pharmacological therapy provides the best results. Chronic disease management is important for minimization of episodes of relapse and their impact. Treatment of addiction saves lives.

Addiction professionals and persons in recovery know the hope that is found in recovery. Recovery is available even to persons who may not at first be able to perceive this hope, especially when the focus is on linking the health consequences to the disease of addiction. **As in other health conditions, self-management, with mutual support, is very important in recovery from addiction**. Peer support such as that found in various "self-help" activities is beneficial in optimizing health status and functional outcomes in recovery.

Recovery from addiction is best achieved through a combination of self-management, mutual support, and professional care provided by trained and certified professionals.

Appendix B: Journaling Template

Keep it Simple

Journal writing at its core is simple. Write quickly, as this frees your brain from 'shoulds' and other blocks to successful journaling. Begin anywhere, and don't worry about spelling and punctuation. If it helps, pick a theme for the day, week, or month (for example, peace of mind, confusion, change, or anger). The most important rule is that there are no rules.

Keep it private

Privacy is key if you are to write without censor, which is essential to the process. Your journal is a safe place for you to explore whatever is on your mind without worrying about how it will affect anyone else. If you fear it will be read, you'll censor yourself and the benefits of journaling will be lost.

Do it frequently

Daily journaling for approximately twenty minutes provides the most benefits and the best results. If you only write when you feel you need to, you will always be in crisis management and you'll continue to live in reactionary mode. The benefit of frequent journaling is that it helps you recognize patterns in your life, helps you gain perspective and more awareness. If you're unable to journal every day, do it as often as you can. A couple times a week is better than not at all. If you miss some time, just get back to it without beating yourself up.

Which medium to choose?

Once you have decided to keep a journal, your next decision is the medium to use for it. There are plenty of options and what works for one person may not work for another. Many recommend keeping a paper journal because writing by hand uses a different part of your brain than typing does. People tend to write slower than typing so it allows more time for reflection. If writing in a journal is not the preferable option to you, go ahead and use a computer, but keep in mind that the more you automate the process, the less you are actually journaling, so you do not get quite the same benefits.

Appendix C: List of Feelings

Happy	Fear	Joy	Content
Frustration	Irritable	Love	Peace
Greed	Lust	Jealousy	Affection
Loss	Ignorant	Envy	Shame
Grief	Stupid	Satisfied	Vengeful
Anger	Useless	Worried	Claustrophobic
Sadness	Wasteful	Prideful	Trapped
Depressed	Achieved	Empathy	Abnormal
Anxious	Interested	Ecstasy	Unusual
Stress	Eager	Judgmental	Amused
Overwhelmed	Virtuous	Compassion	Abandoned
Confused	Worried	Equanimity	Searching
Tense	Helpless	Relieved	Seeking
Scared	Ambitious	Balanced	Euphoric
Desiring	Cynical	Guilty	Restless
Craving	Threatened	Fulfilled	Bewildered
Empty	Generous	Weak	Centred
Blue	Lonely	Energized	Whole
Cheerful	Satisfied	Giddy	Fragmented
Fatigue	Gentle	Tired	Broken
Surrender	Fragile	Delight	Aware
Hope	Careful	Pleasure	Spiritual

Faith	Distracted	Rejected	Egotistic
Confident	Disappointed	Relief	Small
Cautious	Dissatisfied	Pressure	Inspired
Hesitant	Apathy	Controlled	Alert
Strong	Sorry	Controlling	Astounded
Nurturing	Forgiving	Inauthentic	Awe
Caring	Resentment	Deprived	Foolish
Comfortable	Disgust	Discomfort	Glad
Stuffed	Playful	High	Glee
Authentic	Lost	Connected	Bored
Disenchanted	Frazzled	Manipulated	Tired
Kind	Aroused	Flat	Childish
Grace	Terrified	Deceived	Valued
Placid	Rage	Betrayed	Ambivalent
Calm	Numb	Forced	Engaged
Attentive	Nervous	Coerced	Betrayed
Aware	Silly	Victim	Pity
Aggressive	Hostile	Regret	Adamant
Bitchy	Competitive	Hopeless	Lazy
Destructive	Isolated	Pain	Panicked
Deceitful	Precarious	Shy	Solemn

Appendix D: Chakras

OUR PHYSICAL BODY, ENERGY BODY, AND THE CHAKRA SYSTEM

As much as people are familiar with their physical body and we have talked a lot about the brain in this book, there is an energy field within and around our bodies that is not understood by Western medicine. The Vedic system of knowledge from ancient India recognizes the existence of a subtle (energy) body that affects the functions of our physical body in various ways. The chakra system is a way of understanding that connection in a practical way for health.

Chakra is a Sanskrit word meaning "wheel" or "turning". Chakras are energy centres in our subtle body in which energy flows. There are many chakras in the subtle human body but there are seven that are considered the most important. The seven main chakras are located along the spine, extending out the front and back of the body. Each chakra has a number of specific qualities that correspond to the refinement of energy from the base-level material self-identity, located at the first chakras, up to the higher vibration spirit-level awareness of being at our crown (head). Chakras take up and collect prana (life force energy), and transform and pass on energy. Each chakra is associated with a certain part of the body and a certain organ, which it provides with the energy it needs to function. Additionally, just as every organ in the human body has its equivalent on the mental and spiritual level, so too every chakra corresponds to a specific aspect of human behaviour and development. Our circular spirals of energy differ in size and activity from person to person. They vibrate at different levels relative to the awareness of the individual and their ability to integrate the characteristics of each into their life. The lower chakras are associated with fundamental emotions and needs, for the energy here vibrates at a lower frequency and is therefore denser in nature. The finer energies of the upper chakras correspond to our higher mental and spiritual aspirations and faculties.

The openness and flow of energy through our chakras determines our state of health and balance. Knowledge of our more subtle energy system empowers us to maintain balance and harmony on the physical, social, mental, and spiritual level. All meditation and yoga systems seek to balance out the energy of the chakras by purifying the lower energies and guiding them upwards. Through the use of grounding and living consciously with an awareness of how you acquire and spend energy, you become capable of balancing your life force with your mental, physical, social, and spiritual self.

Each center has an integral function in creating our energetic balance. It is through the study of our energetic and physical being that people can create health, emotional stability, and spiritual bliss. Blocked energy in any one or more of the seven chakras can often lead to illness, so it is important to understand what each chakra represents and what you can do to keep this energy flowing freely.

1. ROOT CHAKRA — Represents our foundation and feeling of being grounded.

- Location: Base of spine in tailbone area.

- Emotional issues: Survival issues such as financial independence, money, and food.

- Fear can create a block here.

2. SACRAL CHAKRA — Our connection and ability to accept others and new experiences.

- Location: Lower abdomen, about two inches below the navel and two inches in (Also called the Spleen Chakra).

- Emotional issues: Sense of abundance, well-being, pleasure, sexuality.

- Anger and resentment can create a block here.

3. SOLAR PLEXUS CHAKRA — Our ability to be confident and in-control of our lives.

- Location: Upper abdomen in the stomach area.

- Emotional issues: Self-worth, self-confidence, self-esteem.

- Shame can create a block here.

4. HEART CHAKRA — Our ability to love.

- Location: Center of chest just above heart.

- Emotional issues: Love, joy, inner peace.

- Inability to connect with feelings or lack of boundaries with feelings of others can create problems here.

5. THROAT CHAKRA — Our ability to communicate.

- Location: Throat.

- Emotional issues: Communication, self-expression of feelings, our truth.

- Lack of honesty in communication can create a block here.

6. THIRD EYE CHAKRA — Our ability to focus on and see the big picture.

- Location: Forehead between the eyes (Also called the Brow Chakra).

- Emotional issues: Intuition, imagination, wisdom, ability to think and make decisions.

- Lack of ability to consider what is beyond our immediate perception with our five senses—hearing, touch, vision, taste, and smell—can create a block here.

7. CROWN CHAKRA — The highest chakra represents our ability to be fully connected spiritually.

- Location: The very top of the head.

- Emotional issues: Inner and outer beauty, our connection to spirituality, pure bliss.

- Lack of ability to connect with ourselves, others, and our higher power at a spiritual/consciousness level can create a block here.

Appendix E: Sample Recovery Schedule

Time	Monday	Tuesday	Wednesday
6:30-8:30am	Wake-up, meditate, morning reading, get ready, eat breakfast	Wake-up, meditate, morning reading, get ready, eat breakfast	Wake-up, meditate, morning reading, get ready, eat breakfast
8:30-12:00pm	Work	Work	Work
12:00-1:00pm	Lunch, walk outside	Lunch, yoga class	Lunch
1:00-5:00pm	Work-break for snack, walk around mid-afternoon	Work-break for snack, walk around mid-afternoon	Work-break for snack, walk around mid-afternoon
5:00-6:00pm	Come home, meditate, prepare and eat dinner,	Come home, meditate, prepare and eat dinner	Come home, meditate, prepare and eat dinner
6:00-7:00pm	Relax, read/watch TV, prepare lunch for tomorrow	Relax, read/watch TV, prepare lunch for tomorrow	Relax, read/watch TV, prepare lunch for tomorrow
7:00-9:00pm	Go to 12-step meeting	Stay home, relax, do stretching	Go to the gym, relax
9:00-10:00pm	Bedtime ritual: journal feelings, read, pray	Bedtime ritual: journal feelings, read, pray	Bedtime ritual: journal feelings, read, pray
10:00pm	Bedtime	Bedtime	Bedtime

Thursday	Friday	Saturday	Sunday
Wake-up, meditate, morning reading, get ready, eat breakfast	Wake-up, meditate, morning reading, get ready, eat breakfast	Wake-up, meditate, morning reading, get ready, eat breakfast	Wake-up, meditate, morning reading, get ready, eat breakfast
Work	Work	Walk, go to a 12-step meeting	Go to church
Lunch, go for a walk	Lunch	Lunch out after meeting	Lunch at home
Work-break for snack, walk around mid-afternoon	Work-break for snack, walk around mid-afternoon	Fun! (Art class, physical activity, movie, etc.)	Relax at home- clean, read, cook
Come home, meditate, prepare and eat dinner	Come home, meditate, prepare and eat dinner	Prepare and eat dinner	Cook dinner for guests
Relax, read/ watch TV, prepare lunch for tomorrow	Relax, read/ watch TV	Relax at home or go out with people who are healthy for me	Relax, read/ watch TV, prepare lunch for tomorrow
Group therapy	Go to 12-step meeting	Keep enjoying my evening	Physical activity
Bedtime ritual: journal feelings, read, pray	Bedtime ritual: journal feelings, read, pray	Bedtime ritual: journal feelings, read, pray	Bedtime ritual: journal feelings, read, pray
Bedtime	Bedtime	Bedtime	Bedtime

Appendix F: My Recovery Schedule Template

Time	Monday	Tuesday	Wednesday
6:30-8:30am			
8:30-12:00pm			
12:00-1:00pm			
1:00-5:00pm			
5:00-6:00pm			
6:00-7:00pm			
7:00-9:00pm			
9:00-10:00pm			
10:00pm			

Thursday	Friday	Saturday	Sunday

End Notes

Introduction

1. Dr. Daniel Amen has been a leader in imaging and identifying problems in different areas of the brain and correlating them with mental health problems and pathological behaviours. He is a double board-certified psychiatrist, teacher, *New York Times* best-selling author, including *Change Your Brain, Change Your Life*. Amen is the founder and medical director of the Amen Clinics in the USA.

Chapter One

1. The research around Addiction as a problem with the brain goes back many decades. The National Institute of Drug Abuse (NIDA) has been the biggest agency sponsoring research in this area around the world. Alan Leshner, director of NIDA in the 1990s, made a very strong effort to publicize that Addiction is a brain disease. Bob Dupont was the first director of NIDA (1973-78) and the second "drug czar" (1973-77), the title associated with the position of director of the Office of National Drug Control Policy, under Presidents Nixon and Ford. Bob Dupont's book *The Selfish Brain*, published in 2000, remains a masterpiece in understanding some of the basic concepts. The current director of NIDA is Nora Volkow, who is an amazing neuroscientist, and continues to move forward in helping us understand how the brain is affected by Addiction, beyond the effect of substances. Historical and current references can be found by searching on the internet about Drs. DuPont, Leshner, Volkow, and NIDA in general.

2. The two neurobiologists who have worked tirelessly in improving our understanding of brain dysfunction in Addiction are Drs. Eliot Gardner and George Koob. Searching under these names would bring interested readers to much more historical and current information.

3. Drs. Eric Nestler and Robert Malenka published a very important article in *Scientific American* in March 2004 that highlights the common Addiction circuitry, where they emphasize that it is important to appreciate the changed architecture of the brain, in addition to dysfunction at the molecular level. Their article can be accessed at http://www.scientificamerican.com/article/the-addicted-brain/ These leaders, together with another colleague, Dr. Steve Hyman, continue to shine a light on Addiction and mental health problems, especially depression and anhedonia, which refers to the increasing inability to find any pleasure even in things that would be pleasurable.

4. Dr. Ken Blum has been a leader in genetic research and has translated the dopaminergic system related research into a unifying concept called the Reward Deficiency Syndrome (Blum K, Oscar-Berman, M, Jacobs W, McLaughlin T, Gold M., 2014 - *see Bibliography*). He is also the Editor-in-Chief of Journal of Reward Deficiency Syndrome that has a seminal article about the neurobiology of Addiction and recovery (Blum K, Badgaiyan RD, Agan G, Fratantonio J, Simpatico T, et al. 2015 - *see Bibliography*)

5. More information about diabetes as a chronic disease is available through the American Diabetes Association: www.diabetes.org

6. Drs. Howard Edenberg and Kenneth Kendler have done and presented extensive research that has established that the heritability of substance-related disorders is 50-60%. This has profound implications for children who have one or both parents affected by the disease of Addiction. The inheritability percentage goes up depending on how the genetic inheritance (chromosomes) from both parents is combined in each child that can vary the expression of the disease of Addiction.

7. There is growing amount of knowledge related to epigenetics, which is the science of genetic expression and factors that affect the expression through exposure to chemicals and environment, together with changing the expression through alternatives in thoughts and environment. Two YouTube videos of note are:

Dr. Eric Nestler:
https://www.youtube.com/watch?v=Dx_H01XY5BY
and Dr. Bruce Lipton:
https://www.youtube.com/watch?v=kqG5TagD0uU

Genes are a blueprint and the expression of genes can be affected by various environmental factors. Individual perceptions and interpretation of internal and external stimuli can affect how the brain dysfunctions or functions.

Chapter Two

1. Decades of scientific research have clearly established now that Addiction is a brain disease. This is not just a theory. It is an explanation of how the brain works and influences behaviour, together with the effects substances have. The NIDA website (http://www.drugabuse.gov/related-topics/addiction-science) offers more explanations to help people appreciate the complexities in brain responses rather than viewing the substance use or addictive behaviour as "bad" or "immoral" behaviour.

2. Even back in the eighteenth century, there was an appreciation that the problems related to alcoholism went beyond the alcohol as a substance. Dr. Benjamin Rush, a prominent American and a signatory of the American Declaration of Independence, addressed issues related to Addiction and mental health in his book, *Medical Inquiries and Observations upon the Diseases of the Mind*, back in 1784. He coined the term "alcoholic disease syndrome" to capture the complexities of alcoholism. More information

about this is available here: http://www.health.am/psy/more/
dr-benjamin-rush-and-his-views-on-alcoholism/

3. In the nineteenth century, "inebriety" was recognized by some
as a disease and "alcohol and opiate (drug) addiction" were conceptualized as the manifestation. The Journal of Inebriety chronicles the
thinking of the time as the focus was more on complications as the
understanding of Addiction as a brain disease was elusive.

4. The establishment of Alcoholics Anonymous in the 1930s led
to more discussion of alcoholism as a disease characterized by loss
of control over alcohol use and over one's life, with alcoholism being
described in *The Big Book* (1939) as an "obsession of the mind" (p. 23)
and a "physical allergy of the body" (p. xxviii). These ideas were proposed by Dr. William Silkworth and remain part of the AA *Big Book*
as 'The Doctor's Opinion'. Dr. E.M. "Bunky" Jellinek (1890-1963)
was an American physician whose early career took him to Europe
and Africa began to study alcoholism and its complications after his
return to Yale in the 1930s. He published his book *Alcohol Addiction
and Chronic Alcoholism* in 1942. He moved to Europe again in the
1950s to work with the World Health Organization. His best known
work, *The Disease Concept of Alcoholism* (1960), was published just a
few years before his passing away. More information can be accessed
at http://en.wikipedia.org/wiki/E._Morton_Jellinek

5. The controversies about whether Addiction is a disease or
social problem continues, largely because people, including professionals, do not appreciate the problems in the brain. Changed
behaviour in the context of controlling or stopping substance use
remains a standard for success; and disappointment follows with
blaming the individual and/or treatment centre for relapse, which is
part of inadequately treated disease. In India, the prevalent terminology in treatment has been "de-addiction" as highlighted on this
website http://deaddictioncentres.in/ "De-addiction" usually focuses
solely on solving the addiction problem by stopping the behaviours,
treating withdrawal if one has to, and to consider the problem solved

until the inevitable relapse happens, thus calling it "re-addiction" if things turn out of control.

6. The World Health Organization (WHO), part of the UN system, acknowledged difficulties in developing a definition of addiction in its report in 1952. More details are available in this report: World Health Organization Expert Committee on Drugs Liable to Produce Addiction. *Third report*. Geneva, Switzerland: WHO, 1952. By the 1960s, there was an increasing consensus within the WHO to drop the terms "habituation" and "addiction" in favor of the term "drug dependence" because it was thought that there was too much stigma connected with the term "addiction". Unfortunately, the stigma has not gone away and more confusion has resulted because for some "dependence" and "addiction" are synonymous, whereas others consider "dependence" as a medical or psychiatric issue in contrast to "addiction" that may be bad behaviour.

7. Research on the reward circuitry has revealed that dopamine surges in the brain for all humans are normally driven by food and sex with a feedback mechanism of satiation, which says 'enough'. However, with those who have Addiction the same circuit becomes associated with saying 'more'. The following websites explore the brain disease concepts from a more practical perspective: http://www.famh.ca and http://www.attcnetwork.org/explore/priorityareas/science/disease/

8. The DSM is in its current fifth edition, called DSM 5. Published by the American Psychiatric Association, it classifies mental disorders in the context of behavioural checklists. It uses the term disorder rather than disease. An assumption is also made that the disorder is cured or in remission if the criteria that were once met are no longer met in the affected person's behaviours. More information about the DSM is available at http://www.dsm5.org

9. The definition of Addiction and other related terminology has been established by review of research and clinical experience by senior Addiction medicine physicians and extensive consultation with various stakeholders via the American Society of Addiction

Medicine (ASAM). More information about the Addiction Medicine medical societies is available on their websites: http://www.asam. org, http://www.csam.org and http://www.isamweb.org

10. This is the correlation with "powerlessness" over Addiction and "unmanageability" of life, as is described in step one of 12-step programs. Powerlessness does not mean helplessness rather surrender and acceptance regarding something that is not in one's control. Addiction is a disease that has an automaticity that is not controllable. The more one tries to control, the more the disease goes out of control making the affected person's life unmanageable, together with having an adverse impact on friends and family relationships.

11. Cravings can be viewed as intense memories that draw people back to using or they represent withdrawal symptoms that are triggered by the environment. Brain imaging studies have also shown some intense brain activation when pictures that are linked to drug use (like a pipe, or a white powdery substance resembling cocaine) are shown to people with Addiction. More information about this is available at the NIH website: http://www.ncbi.nlm.nih.gov/pmc/articles/PMC2978100/

Chapter Three

1. More information about Alcoholics Anonymous' "stinking thinking" is available at http://stinkin-thinkin.com/2009/04/27/stinking-thinking/

Around 1983, Dr. David Sedlak described addictive thinking as a "person's inability to make consistently healthy decisions on his or her own behalf". Dr. Abraham Twerski has written extensively about addictive thinking and dysfunctional emotional responses of people with Addiction. These can vary from no reaction in a circumstance that would elicit a significant response, e.g. maintaining a stoic appearance despite having lost a close family member to death; or a strong emotional reaction when an average person may take it in a stride, e.g. a friend not acknowledging a greeting because s/he is preoccupied is interpreted by someone with Addiction as a deliberate slight, around which a whole script of paranoia and resentments may emerge.

2. Journaling allows an individual to document their thoughts and feelings without judgment. Further, it usually results in more clarity as the individual can reflect on what came out during the process of honest expression. Scientific evidence supports the notion that journaling has a positive impact on overall well-being. The PsychCentral website http://psychcentral.com/lib/the-health-benefits-of-journaling/000721 explores the benefits. This link, http://www.appleseeds.org/100 Journaling.htm has listed a hundred benefits of it.

3. Relaxation techniques can vary from simple, sequential tightening and relaxing of muscles all over one's body to focused, deep breathing to visualization and guided imagery to achieve a quietening of the mind and shift away from worries and uncomfortable feelings. The following website offers some more explanations and suggestions to try out: http://www.stress-relief-tools.com/visualization-relaxation.html

4. Meditation does not mean clearing your mind, as many people commonly assert. A definition of meditation is available from the Free Dictionary at http://medical-dictionary.thefreedictionary.com/meditation that describes various ideas that fall under the broad umbrella of meditation in common understanding today. True meditation is a mental technique or discipline by which the individual moves beyond the thinking mind into a deeper, more profound state of awareness and transcendental state. With meditation, one achieves better self–knowledge, clarity of thought, lowered stress, improved health, greater focus, and overall wellbeing without making much effort. Transcendental meditation (TM) is a specific mental technique that has been validated as being beneficial with extensive research. More information at http://www.tm.org

5. The Johari Window was developed and published first by Luft & Ingham in the 1950s. More information about the Johari Window is readily available on the internet. For those more interested, the

Wikipedia article may be a place to start further exploration: http://en.wikipedia.org/wiki/Johari_window

6. Self-talk is closely connected with behaviours, as the thoughts and feelings that drive self-talk also affect what behaviours may or may not follow. Hence, unhealthy self-talk usually contributes to problem behaviours continuing whereas healthy self-talk can lead to behaviour change towards better health. The challenge is to cultivate awareness of how it is affecting you, your actions, and others around you. There are numerous books written about self-talk, implications, and the 'how-to' of making change. *Choicemaking* by Sharon Wegsheider-Cruse (1986) and *Addictive Thinking* by Abraham Twerski (1997) are two useful books that explore these concepts in the context of appreciating that negative self-talk is a barrier to change, while encouraging more awareness and positive self-talk for healthier behaviours.

Chapter Four

1. The American Psychological Association's (APA) *Dictionary of Psychology* documents the consensus definitions related to terms commonly used in psychology, in an attempt to increase awareness, understanding, and clarity related to our internal human experience. The APA website offers more information for those looking for more precision in psychological terminology: http://www.apa.org/pubs/books/4311007.aspx

2. The 'dry drunk' syndrome is described in the *Big Book of Alcoholics Anonymous* as feeling "irritable, restless and discontented". This relates to the dysfunctional response of the definition of Addiction and can be very problematic if one is not aware of it oneself and is not taking recovery action to deal with feelings. This website offers some more information of feelings and behaviours that are associated with the 'dry drunk': http://addictionrecoverybasics.com/what-is-a-dry-drunk/

3. Brene Brown (2007, 2009, 2010) is a research professor at the University of Houston, who has spent years studying shame, as

well as vulnerability, resilience, and worthiness. She distinguishes between shame, humiliation, embarrassment, and guilt as follows: "Shame is the intensely painful feeling or experience that we are flawed and therefore unworthy of connection or belonging" (2009, p. 42). Humiliation does not feel deserved, whereas shame does because there is a part of our brain telling us 'you are not worthy'. Embarrassment involves intense discomfort with oneself and is often experienced upon having a socially unacceptable act witnessed by or revealed to others. It is similar to shame, except that shame may be experienced for an act known only by the self. Also, embarrassment can be humorous and fleeting, whereas shame can be devastating and perpetual (Brown, 2009, p. 43).

4. The chakra system is part of the Vedic knowledge from ancient India that posits energy nodes in the body that connect with physicality. It is described in more detail in Appendix D.

5. The 'type A personality' was first described in the 1950s as having a strong association with high blood pressure and heart disease. Over the years, health care providers have come to appreciate that the strong drive to prove one self or seek approval from others by doing is more likely than not connected with a deep sense of shame related to not feeling good enough, while seeking external validation from achievements and/or positive strokes from others. In psychiatric terminology, avoidant personality disorder is associated with shame, where the incessant actions are a way to avoid dealing with emotions and feelings that may be perceived to be problematic. The 'type A personality' is sometimes associated with narcissism and grandiosity, which is again a cover for shame. However, it is important to appreciate that all of these are manifestations of the disease of Addiction that is characterized by avoidance, escape, and isolation.

6. Pride refers to an inflated sense of self, status, and accomplishments. It can be a cover for shame such that a certain accomplishment or status establishes an image to counter the not feeling good enough.

7. Grandiosity refers to a sense of superiority compared to others that is usually not based in reality. It often involves over-inflation of one's own capacities, while downplaying others.

8. Resentment means feeling repeatedly. Although usually associated with anger or frustration, it can be felt through a myriad of feelings, which can come from fear and shame too. A Step 4 inventory allows one to examine feelings much more honestly and closely so that they do not continue to fester by trapping people in a victim role.

Chapter Five

1. Ask, Advise, Assess, Assist, Arrange are common parts of these techniques that refer to providing guidance to achieve lasting behaviour change for smoking cessation. The following link provides more information for those interested: http://www.ahrq.gov/professionals/clinicians-providers/guidelines-recommendations/tobacco/5steps.html

The principles are applicable to behaviour change in general. However, it must be appreciated that when Addiction is present, the assessment needs to be more comprehensive along biological, psychological, social, and spiritual dimensions, and more professional, directive assistance needs to be provided with or without arranging a referral to more specialized resources.

2. The following link to the Mayo Clinic site provides a list of complications that can occur due to tobacco use: http://www.mayoclinic.org/diseases-conditions/nicotine-dependence/basics/complications/con-20014452

This site also provides more information about medical complications due to other substances. Extensive medical complications information regarding Addiction and mental health problems is available at the website for the Centre for Addiction and Mental Health in Toronto, Canada: http://www.camh.ca/en/hospital/health_information/a_z_mental_health_and_addiction_information/Pages/default.aspx

3. National Institute on Drug Abuse remains the biggest funding resource for addiction-related research around the world and their website offers a wealth of information –

http://www.drugabuse.gov/

4. The term immunotherapy refers to vaccines that are being developed for nicotine, cocaine, and methamphetamines such that the immune response would sequester the drug in a vaccinated individual, rendering the drug ineffective on the brain. Most of these research projects are being supported by the American National Institute on Drug Abuse (NIDA).

5. Ongoing research is documenting the presence/co-occurrence of alcohol-related problems and other compulsive behaviours such as sexual acting out or gambling. The following link provides more information about this. This website provides links to other articles related to Addiction and its complications: http://www.sciencedirect.com/science/article/pii/S0376871614020080

6. The discovery of the cannabinoid receptor in the early 1990s has led to many advances related to the endo-cannabinoid circuitry that keeps us well, with problems resulting when it is compromised due to internal circuitry problems or by the use of marijuana from the outside. The National Institute of Health is a good source for articles such as for those wanting to explore the research advances in this area. For example: http://www.ncbi.nlm.nih.gov/pmc/articles/PMC3267552/

7. The following link to NIDA resources has good factual information related to inhalants and related problems, especially the association with alcohol and tobacco use: http://www.drugabuse.gov/publications/research-reports/inhalants/what-are-inhalants

8. This link will take you to a current article that discusses this phenomenon of chasing from the perspective of research evidence: http://www.sciencedirect.com/science/article/pii/S0191886999000525

9. The Mayo Clinic offers a nice explanation of various types of bariatric surgery and the rationale for them: http://www.

mayoclinic.org/tests-procedures/bariatric-surgery/in-depth/
weight-loss-surgery/ART-20045334?pg=2

10. The fellowship of Anorexics and Bulimics Anonymous (ABA) began around 1992 and continues to grow in various parts of the world: http://aba12steps.org/

11. The s-fellowships include Sexaholics Anonymous (SA) (www.sa.org), Sex Addicts Anonymous (SAA) (www.saa-recovery.org) and Sex and Love Addicts Anonymous (SLAA) (www.slaafws.org).

12. Borderline Personality Disorder is considered a psychiatric diagnosis as discussed at www.nimh.nih.gov/health/topics/borderline-personality-disorder/index.shtml. However, the relationship problems and related cognitive distortions fit the framework of Addiction involving relationships. This is important as recovery offers much more hope in context of Addiction, whereas trying to change behaviour alone can be much more problematic and hopeless.

13. A quick search on the internet will reveal a variety of definitions for codependence, which have some common features but conceptualizations differ. The 12-step fellowship called CoDA (Codependents Anonymous — www.coda.org) is a reasonable place to start for some basic information. However, problems persist if people approach it as being something different than Addiction involving relationships, especially if the individual continues to engaging in ongoing substance use, while trying to change in context of relationships.

14. Dr. Stephen B. Karpman has done pioneering work in this area and his website offers extensive information about his concepts. We have adapted his ideas in a very practical way in our book and practice to define problems in relationships and offer a framework for solutions. http://karpmandramatriangle.com/

15. Dr. Nora Volkow, Director of National Institute on Drug Abuse (NIDA) has done the research that has led to the development of the following diagram to illustrate the brain circuitry differences between (a) non-addicted brains and (b) addicted brains. Saliency refers to the attractiveness or importance given to a

substance or behaviour that the brain is contemplating for engagement. Distortions in memory in context of the salience further over-riding the impairment in control contribute to impulsiveness and compulsion.

Chapter Six

1. The fellowship of Alcoholics Anonymous (www.aa.org) has been providing extensive peer support for over eight decades now. Peers in recovery are able to listen to struggles, cravings, relationship issues, frustrations, and emotions that come up with an authentic reality that others who do not struggle with Addiction or have not acknowledged their Addiction cannot. Here the person in recovery finds love and acceptance that they may not have experienced elsewhere. While Addiction was primarily perceived as a moral failing, there were those at the time, including one of Bill W's treating practitioners, Dr. William Silkworth. Dr. Silkworth believed that alcoholism came with it a mental obsession and "allergy" towards alcohol that he documented in 'The Doctor's Opinion' at the beginning of the *Big Book* of AA. Dr. Silkworth's perspective was more accurately aligned with what is known about Addiction today and viewed it as an illness, rather than 'bad people making bad choices'. Dr. Silkworth also highlighted the need for abstinence as a foundation for recovery. Although it is now known that allergy is a problem related to the immune system, Dr. Silkworth's description of "allergy" was not connected with the immune system. It must be appreciated that the context in which this idea was generated makes it a valid one for the time; that is, that the brain and body of someone with Addiction reacts differently to alcohol, just as an allergy represents a pathological response in only those that are sensitive to that substance.

2. There continues to be an overwhelming resistance and reluctance amongst health care providers to bring up the topic of spirituality, yet it is a critical foundation for healthy recovery, as evidenced by the 12-step programs. These programs are undoubtedly the most

effective ways to achieve and maintain sobriety (Vaillant, 2005 - *see Bibliography*).

3. In active Addiction, goals and priorities become skewed to substance/problem behaviour pursuit and use. A helpful tool for goal setting is SMART (Doran, 1981 - *see Bibliography*). This means making goals: specific, measurable, attainable, realistic, and time-specific.

4. It is essential that the stages of change (Prochaska & DiClemente, 2005 - *see Bibliography*) be kept in mind during assessment and treatment such that the individuals can be approached at the stage where they are at. The model proposes five stages of change: pre-contemplation, contemplation, preparation, action, and maintenance. Each of these stages is designed for people to be able to determine how ready somebody is to make a change in their life. Relapse is sometimes identified as a sixth stage, however, it is better conceptualized as a process in which the individual goes back to contemplation or pre-contemplation, such that substance use or engagement in addictive behaviours resumes.

5. PAWS is an acronym for post-acute-withdrawal syndrome and is also sometimes called protracted withdrawal syndrome. Symptoms are usually triggered by labile mood states and/or stressors/stimuli in the external environment that trigger a strong response that is dysfunctional and often produces physiological symptoms that are dysphoric to the individual. PAWS is usually more common in the first two years of recovery, which characterize the action stage of change, but can be triggered at any time because of the disease of Addiction affecting memory circuitry. The following websites offer some more information that may be helpful in understanding:

http://www.recoveryfirst.org/the-symptoms-of-post-acute-withdrawal-syndrome.html/ and http://addictionsandrecovery.org/post-acute-withdrawal.htm

Chapter Seven

1. Roles in an alcoholic/addictive family have been classified as the person with Addiction, chief enabler, hero, scapegoat, clown,

and wallflower. More information is available from the following sources: http://www.smcok.com/media/newspaper...lic_family.htm, Children of Alcoholics; This Is A War — ADDICTION, and Alcoholic Family Roles Alcohol Self-Help News

2. The setting of boundaries requires a lot of practice. Some practical guidance related to healthy vs. unhealthy is available at website for the Center for Human Potential http://www.yourpotential. net/3/5/A Checklist on Boundaries in a Relationship.html

3. Non-verbal communication is discussed by Barker & Rouch Gaut, 2002 (*see Bibliography*).

4. As much as people classify communication styles in a variety of ways, it is useful to appreciate the four common styles of verbal communication: passive, passive-aggressive, aggressive, and assertive. The following resource offers a nice framework: http://marcimentalhealthmore.com/2013/09/04/resource-communication-styles/communication-styles/

Chapter Eight

1. National organizations such as Canadian Centre on Substance Abuse (www.ccsa.ca) and National Institute on Drug Abuse (www.drugabuse.gov) have produced many documents to guide treatment for substance use disorders. Unfortunately, many research and treatment guidelines retain a substance-specific focus, which continues to reinforce the notion that treatment involves stopping or controlling substance use.

2. Psychosocial rehabilitation is also sometimes called the Minnesota model because Hazelden (www.hazelden.org), which traces its origins to 1949, began treating alcoholics in a structured fashion, utilizing the twelve steps of Alcoholics Anonymous. This can be considered the beginning of the therapeutic technique called Twelve Step Facilitation when it is delivered by a qualified professional. Dr. Gordon Bell, a physician in Toronto, began treating alcoholics in his own home in the 1940s. He developed a treatment model that also utilized twelve steps and disulfiram. This grew into

the standard of treatment at the Donwood Institute in 1967 that has now been incorporated into the Centre for Addiction and Mental Health (www.camh.ca) in Toronto. The program that focused on physical-psychological-social rehabilitation is described in Dr. Bell's book (Bell, 1970). The American Society of Addiction Medicine (www.asam.org) has produced public policy statements on treatment.

3. The ASAM Criteria Text (Mee-Lee, 2013) has been developed to provide guidance for treatment of Addiction, substance-related and co-occurring conditions. It provides detailed guidance for assessment and treatment. It is rapidly becoming the definitive reference guide for assessment and evaluating treatment progress.

4. Opioids are commonly taken by people for pain relief on acute and chronic bases. In Canada, 8 mg of codeine is formulated with acetaminophen or ASA, which is available without a prescription. There has been a tendency for people to think that taking opioids for pain is somehow different than when taken as an 'escape' or 'recreationally'. Addiction is often not recognized until aberrant behaviour becomes so evident that the presence of pain or not does not matter; and pain and Addiction treatment both become very challenging. The following link has a relevant article on this subject that reviews the evidence for long term opioid use for pain: http://www.ncbi.nlm.nih.gov/pmc/articles/PMC3590544/

The risk for anyone prescribed opioids needs to be evaluated carefully. The following link also provides useful guidance: http://www.opioidrisk.com/node/709

5. Research related to pharmacotherapy for craving is ongoing. The most efficacious data is available for naltrexone. The following website connected to the National Institutes of Health provides some credible information for drugs one may want to look up http://www.nlm.nih.gov/medlineplus/

6. Anti-depressants have become one of the most widely prescribed medications in North America, while the data for their effectiveness remains elusive and the risks, especially of suicide and other side-effects or complications, remain significant. The following

article offers some perspective: http://www.ncbi.nlm.nih.gov/pmc/articles/PMC558707/

7. ASAM established a Descriptive and Diagnostic Terminology Action Group (DDTAG) around 2007, which has produced the definition of addiction and other related terminology. The work is ongoing and information is available at www.asam.org under the policy tab.

8. Cognitive-Behavioural Therapy (CBT) was developed by Dr. Aaron Beck in the 1960s and has continued to evolve since then (Beck & Beck, 2011). CBT has become one of the most common psychotherapeutic approaches for various mental health issues, including depression, anxiety, anxiety-related disorders (e.g., obsessive-compulsive disorder, phobias, and post-traumatic stress disorder), as well as Addiction specifically related to drugs, alcohol, and food/eating disorders (Beck, Wright, Newman, & Liese, 1993).

9. Motivational interviewing (MI) was developed in 1983 by William Miller, along with Stephen Rollnick, in relation to their work with problem drinkers (Miller & Rollnick, 2012). It has great utility in engaging people where they are at without judgment. It helps people evaluate their risks and benefits for behaviour change. The more recent accepted definition "...a collaborative, person-centered form of guiding to elicit and strengthen motivation for change" (Miller & Rose, 2009, p. 137) is getting wide attention now as providers appreciate the importance of patient-centred care that is less prescriptive and more collaborative.

10. Dialectical behaviour therapy (DBT) is a form of psychotherapy that was originally developed by Marsha M. Linehan to treat people with borderline personality disorder (BPD) and chronically suicidal individuals (Linehan, 2014). DBT combines standard cognitive-behavioural techniques for emotion regulation and reality-testing with concepts of distress tolerance, acceptance, and mindful awareness largely derived from Buddhist meditative practice, often called 'mindfulness'. More information is available at http://mindfulnesstherapy.org/dbt/

11. Psychotherapy is a therapeutic interaction between a trained professional and a client, patient, family, couple, or group (Yalom, 2002). It involves getting to know the individual(s) and dealing with resistance to change that is mostly based in cognitive and affective distortions. Care is needed to go around the well-established defenses that are hard to deal with even when they are recognized as being dysfunctional.

12. Mandated treatment is considered to be controversial, however, there is extensive research supporting the success in many settings as people do engage once their brain is away from substances. The following link provides credible information from NIDA: http://www.drugabuse.gov/publications/principles-drug-abuse-treatment-criminal-justice-populations/legally-mandated-treatment-effective

13. The genetic risk for the disease of Addiction is worldwide, even though being Irish Catholic is considered high-risk because of the prevalence of excessive drinking in Ireland, historically. Binge drinking is becoming very widespread globally with men and women. This article offers some perspective: http://www.ncbi.nlm.nih.gov/pubmed/22155620. Dr. Twerski's book (Twerski, 1982) is very illustrative for doctors.

14. The Ontario Medical Association Professional Health Program (php.oma.org) is an exemplary program that has now been in operation for close to twenty years under the leadership of Dr. Mike Kaufmann.

15. The American Board of Addiction Medicine (www.abam.net) got established with the help of ASAM around 2007. It is providing necessary leadership and direction in training and certification of physicians for the ultimate benefit to individuals, families, and society as a whole.

16. The International Society of Addiction Medicine (www.isamweb.org) was founded in 1999 and developed an examination that was first implemented in 2005. There are close links between

the Canadian Society of Addiction Medicine (www.csam.org), ASAM, ABAM and ISAM.

17. The Physician Consortium for Performance Improvement is an initiative of AMA: https://www.ama-assn.org/ama/pub/physician-resources/physician-consortium-performance-improvement.page

It is a physician-led program to identify evidence-based performance measures that are also clinically meaningful to enhance quality in patient care and safety, especially in the context of balancing benefits with potential harms.

Chapter Nine

1. In her book, *When Society Becomes An Addict*, Schaef (1987) explores the idea of how our society has been developing into a closed system, where true choices to individuals are few, as marketing and other pressures herd people into directions that are not necessarily in their best interest nor are they in the best interest of society. She discusses the problems with image management and illusion of control that feed an addictive system.

2. Dr. Bell documents his journey from his childhood to Bellwood (Bell, 1989). He noted, "Our enemy is the most threatening global pandemic that has ever confronted mankind. It is addiction, and I have spent the last forty-two years waging my own campaign against it." Despite the challenges he faced, which were professional and societal, he always took a positive and caring approach to what he called "Operation Survival".

3. The Foundation for Addiction and Mental Health's (www.famh.ca) vision is "a world where addiction and mental health problems are accepted as health conditions, without stigma, where long-term recovery through a continuing care framework and mutual support is available for all". FAMH is also connected with a new mutual support program called RAiAR — Remember Addiction is Addiction Responsible Recovery — which helps people in recovery appreciate the disease of Addiction in its various forms, so that

optimum progress can be made towards holistic recovery, with honesty and humility, boundaries and balance, together with staying in process, with the outcomes being determined by the grace of the higher power.

Glossary

Abdicate. Refuse, disown, reject, abandon.

Abstinence. Intentional and consistent restraint from the pathological pursuit of reward and/or relief that involves the use of substances and other behaviours. These behaviours may involve, but are not necessarily limited to, gambling, video gaming, spending, compulsive eating, compulsive exercise, or compulsive sexual behaviours.

Acceptance and commitment therapy (ACT). A form of clinical behaviour analysis used in psychotherapy. This type of therapy gets its name from one of its core messages, which is 'accept what is out of your personal control and commit to action that improves and enriches your life'. The aim of ACT is to maximize human potential for a rich, full, and meaningful life.

Acute. Having a sudden onset, sharp rise, and short course.

Addiction. Addiction is a primary, chronic disease of brain reward, motivation, memory, and related circuitry. Dysfunction in these circuits leads to characteristic biological, psychological, social, and spiritual manifestations. This is reflected in an individual pathologically pursuing reward and/or relief by substance use and other behaviours.

Addiction is characterized by inability to consistently abstain, impairment in behavioural control, craving, diminished recognition of significant problems with one's behaviours and interpersonal relationships, and a dysfunctional emotional response. Like other chronic diseases, addiction often involves cycles of relapse and remission. Without treatment or engagement in recovery activities, addiction is progressive and can result in disability or premature death.

Addiction Medicine. A medical specialty that deals with the prevention, assessment, and treatment of Addiction

Addictionist. A medical doctor who is additionally certified by the American Society of Addiction Medicine (ASAM) or the American Board of Addiction Medicine (ABAM)

Affective distortions. Exaggerated or distorted feelings.

Agonist maintenance treatment. A treatment option for opioid-dependence (e.g., Methadone). Opioid agonist maintenance therapy may be the primary tool available to engage an opioid-dependent individual in treatment because it relieves unpleasant withdrawal symptoms and cravings associated with abstinence.

Alexithymia. An inability to connect with and describe feelings associated with various emotions.

Allostasis. A resetting of balance or homeostasis in response to stressors that can become pathological.

Amygdala. An almond-shaped structure in the brain; its name comes from the Greek word for "almond". As with most other brain structures, there are two amygdalae in the brain. Each amygdala is located close to the hippocampus, in the frontal portion of the temporal lobe. The amygdala is essential to feel certain feelings and to perceive them in other people. This includes fear and the many changes that it causes in the body.

Anhedonia. The inability to experience pleasure from activities that are normally pleasurable or desirable to promote a sense of well-being. This is a common clinical feature of many mental health problems and is a strong feature of Addiction, especially during acute withdrawal and can be part of the post-acute withdrawal syndrome (PAWS).

Anterior cingulate cortex (ACC). The frontal part of the cingulate cortex. It plays a role in a wide variety of autonomic functions, such as regulating blood pressure and heart rate. It is also involved in rational cognitive functions, such as reward anticipation, decision-making, empathy, impulse control, and emotion.

Attention deficit disorder (ADD). Term used to describe patterns of behaviour that appear most often in school-aged children. Children with these disorders are inattentive, and overly impulsive. They have difficulty sitting still or attending to one thing for a long period, and may seem overactive.

Attention deficit hyperactivity disorder (ADHD). Attention deficit hyperactivity disorder is used to describe patterns of behaviour including being inattentive, overly impulsive and hyperactive. It is the updated term from ADD to include the symptoms associated with hyperactivity.

Barbiturates. A group of drugs in the class known as sedative-hypnotics, which describes their sleep-inducing and anxiety-decreasing effects. Barbiturates can be extremely dangerous because the correct dose is difficult to predict. Even a slight overdose can cause coma or death. Barbiturates are also addictive and can cause a life-threatening withdrawal syndrome.

Basal forebrain. A group of structures that lie near the bottom of the brain in the front of our head. These structures are important in the production of a brain chemical called acetylcholine, which is then distributed widely throughout the brain. Acetylcholine affects the ability of brain cells to transmit information to one another, and encourages plasticity, or learning. Thus, damage to the basal forebrain can reduce the amount of acetylcholine in the brain and impair learning.

Bipolar disorder. Also known as bipolar affective disorder, originally called manic-depressive illness, is described by the American Psychiatric Association as a mental disorder characterized by distinct periods of elevated mood and depression.

Benzodiazepines. A group of drugs that are also called anxiolytics, which means they reduce anxiety. They can also have hypnotic or amnesia-inducing effects. Like alcohol, these drugs increase the efficiency of synaptic transmission of the neurotransmitter GABA by acting on its receptors.

Borderline personality disorder. A mental illness marked by unstable moods, behaviours, and persistent problems in relationships.

Boundaries. By establishing clear personal boundaries, people define themselves in relation to others. To do this, you must be able to identify and respect your values, needs, feelings, opinions, and rights. Boundaries allow people to separate who they are and what they think and feel, from the thoughts and feelings of others.

Buprenorphine. A drug used to treat opioid dependence (opioid drugs, including heroin and narcotic painkillers). Buprenorphine is in a class of medications called opioid partial agonist-antagonists. Buprenorphine alone and the combination of buprenorphine and naloxone (Suboxone) prevent withdrawal symptoms when someone stops taking opioid drugs by producing similar effects to these drugs.

Cannabis. A substance that is commonly known as marijuana.

Cerebrum. The largest and most highly developed part of the human brain. It encompasses about two-thirds of the brain mass and lies over and around most of the structures of the brain. The outer portion of the cerebrum is called the cerebral cortex and is characterized by a layer of tissue called gray matter.

Chakra. The Sanskrit word chakra literally translates to wheel or disk. In yoga, meditation, and Ayurveda, this term refers to wheels of energy throughout the body. There are seven main chakras, which align the spine, starting from the base of the spine through to the crown of the head. To visualize a chakra in the body, imagine a swirling wheel of energy where matter and consciousness meet. This invisible energy, called prana, is vital life force, which keeps us vibrant, healthy, and alive.

Chronic. Persisting for a long time or constantly recurring.

Cingulate cortex. A brain region involved in emotional, cognitive, and motor tasks.

Cingulate gyrus. An important part of the limbic system, the cingulate gyrus helps regulate feelings and pain. It is thought to directly drive the body's conscious response to unpleasant experiences. In addition, it is involved in fear and the prediction (and avoidance) of negative consequences and can help orient the body away from negative stimuli. Also considered the brain's gear shifter, it is responsible for cognitive flexibility, shifting attention, and going from idea to idea.

Codependence. Preoccupation with other peoples thoughts, feelings, and behaviours to the detriment of one's own health.

Cognitive behavioural therapy (CBT) A common type of psychotherapy that helps people understand the relationship between their thoughts, behaviour, physiology, and sometimes feelings.

Cognitive distortions. Exaggerated or irrational thought patterns.

Compulsive. Not able to stop or control doing something.

Contingency management. A strategy used in psychology that seeks to change behaviour by modifying its consequences. It is based upon a simple behavioural principle that if a behaviour is reinforced or rewarded, it is more likely to occur in the future.

Continuing care. Ongoing, long-term support required for those dealing with a chronic disease.

Cortical circuit. Neuron connections in the cortex.

Craving. A state of desire to use substances or engage in addictive behaviours, experienced as a physical or emotional need for reward and/or relief. Craving generally refers to conscious craving, involving subjective awareness of preoccupations or even obsessional thoughts to impulsively or compulsively seek reward and/or relief through substance use and other behaviours. Some have also hypothesized the existence of unconscious craving, in which motivation and drive are increased as part of the neurobiology of addiction. Craving may perpetuate active addiction or lead to relapse in an individual who has been in remission.

Cues. Signal, sign, clue, inkling.

Delirium tremens. Also referred to as DTs, this is an acute episode of delirium that is usually caused by withdrawal from alcohol. It is a very serious form of withdrawal that has a significant degree of mortality associated with it when someone experiences it.

Depressive disorder. Persistent feelings of sadness and worthlessness and a lack of desire to engage in formerly pleasurable activities. It interferes with daily life and normal functioning.

Dialectical behavioural therapy (DBT). A modified form of cognitive-behavioural psychotherapy designed to help people change patterns of behaviours that are not effective and help increase emotional and cognitive regulation.

Disease. An abnormal condition that affects an organ(s) in the body. In humans, disease is often used broadly to refer to any condition that causes pain, dysfunction, distress, social problems, or death to the person afflicted, or similar problems for those in contact with the person. In this broader sense, it sometimes includes injuries, disabilities, disorders, syndromes, infections, isolated symptoms, deviant behaviours, and atypical variations of structure and function. Diseases affect people physically as well as emotionally, as contracting and living with a disease can alter one's perspective on life.

Dopamine. A neurotransmitter that helps control the brain's reward and pleasure centers. Dopamine also helps regulate movement and emotional responses; it enables us not only to see rewards, but to take action to move toward them.

DSM. The abbreviation for the Diagnostic and Statistical Manual of Mental Disorders published by the American Psychiatric Association which offeommon language and standard criteria for the classification of mental disorders.

Dysfunction. Abnormality or impairment. Not working in a healthy manner.

Dysphoric. Generalized feeling of distress.

Empathy. The ability to understand the feelings of another person without taking them on as your own.

Epigenetics. The study of changes in gene activity and how the genome responds to the environment. In order for genes to express themselves or get 'switched on,' environmental factors need to interact with the person's biology, which then affects the extent to which the genetic factors exert their influence.

Generalized anxiety disorder (GAD). A disorder that is characterized by excessive, uncontrollable, and often irrational worry, which reflects apprehensive expectation about events or activities. This excessive worry often interferes with daily functioning,

Grandiosity. An unrealistic sense of superiority, a sustained view of oneself as better than others.

Harm reduction. A treatment and prevention approach that encompasses individual and public health needs, aiming to decrease the health and socio-economic costs and consequences of addiction-related problems, especially medical complications and transmission of infectious diseases, without necessarily requiring abstinence. Abstinence-based treatment approaches are themselves a part of comprehensive harm reduction strategies. A range of recovery activities may be included in every harm reduction strategy.

Hippocampal circuit. Circuitry in the brain region of the hippocampus that is associated with memory.

Holistic. In this context it refers to treatment of the whole person; taking into account biological, psychological, social, and spiritual factors rather than just focusing on the physical symptoms of a disease.

Homeostasis. Any self-regulating process by which biological systems tend to maintain stability while adjusting to conditions that are optimal for survival.

Impulsive. Acting or done without forethought.

Inhibitory. To decrease, suppress, limit, or block the action or function.

Lability. Emotional instability, rapidly changing feelings.

Limbic system. A complex set of structures in the brain that lies on both sides of the thalamus, just under the cerebrum. It includes the hypothalamus, hippocampus, amygdala, and several other nearby areas. The limbic system supports a variety of functions including adrenaline flow, emotion, behaviour, motivation, long-term memory, and sense of smell. Emotional life is largely housed in the limbic system and it has a great deal to do with the formation of memories.

Manifestation. A sign, symptom, indication, evidence, or example.

Medication management. Patient-centred care to optimize safe, effective, and appropriate drug therapy. Care is provided through collaboration with patients and their health care teams.

Methadone. An opioid agonist medication. Methadone reduces withdrawal symptoms and, although developed as a pain reliever, it is now primarily used as part of treatment of Addiction involving opioids for withdrawal management and maintenance.

Morbidity. The occurrence of disease or illness in a person. It is further divided into incidence, the rate of occurrence over a certain period; and prevalence, the numbers of people affected at a given time.

Morphology. A branch of biology that deals with the form and structure of an organism or any of its parts.

Mortality. The relative frequency of deaths in a specific population; death rate is thus described in terms of mortality rates or ratios.

Motivational enhancement therapy. A strategy of therapy that involves a variation of motivational interviewing. The idea of motivational interviewing is based on engaging the client to pursue a behaviour change. The method revolves around goal making, with assistance from the counselor to help guide the client to that specific set goal.

Myriad. Countless, numerous.

Naloxone. An opioid antagonist medication used to counter the effects of opioid overdose.

Network therapy. In using this approach, family and friends are involved in parallel with professional counselling in an effort to bolster therapeutic engagement, provide ongoing support and to promote attitude change.

Neuroadaptation. The process whereby the body compensates for the presence of a chemical in the body so that it can continue to function normally. When neuroadaptation occurs, a person will develop a tolerance and find that they need more of a substance to get the desired effect.

Neurobiology. The study of cells of the nervous system and the organization of these cells into functional circuits that process information and mediate behaviour. It is a sub-discipline of both biology and neuroscience.

Neurochemistry. The specific study of neurochemicals, including neurotransmitters and other molecules that influence the function of neurons.

Neuroscience or Neuroscientific. Any of the sciences, such as neuroanatomy or neurobiology, that deals with the nervous system and its effects on other parts of the body.

Neurotransmission. Also called synaptic transmission, is the process by which signaling molecules called neurotransmitters are released by a neuron (the presynaptic neuron), and bind to and activate the receptors of another neuron (the postsynaptic neuron). Neurotransmission is essential for the process of communication between two neurons.

Nucleus accumbens. Plays a central role in the reward circuit. Its operation is based chiefly on two essential neurotransmitters: dopamine, which promotes desire; and serotonin, whose effects include satiety and inhibition.

Opioids. A family of drugs that have morphine-like effects. The primary medical use for prescription opioids is to relieve pain. They work by binding to opioid receptors in the brain, spinal cord, and other areas of the body. They reduce the sending of pain messages to the brain and reduce feelings of pain.

Opioid Agonist. A drug that acts on the opioid receptor to produce the physiological/chemical effects characteristic of opioids, such as perceptual removal or not caring about pain and other feelings.

Opioid Antagonist. A drug that acts on the opioid receptor to and produces a block or an effect that precipitates withdrawal symptoms. An opioid antagonist produces symptoms that are the opposite of the effects characteristic of opioids.

Pathological. A deviation from normal that contributes to ill health.

Perception. The organization, identification, and interpretation of sensory information in order to represent and understand the environment.

Pharmacotherapy. Therapy or treatment using pharmaceutical drugs.

Post-Acute Withdrawal Syndrome (PAWS). A series of non-specific symptoms in people with Addiction that occur after the acute stage of withdrawal from substances. The symptoms can include persistent fatigue, inability to focus, poor attention span, lack of motivation, irritability, restlessness, discontentedness, nausea, depersonalization, sleep disturbance, or anhedonia. These symptoms can wax and wane in relation to life stressors, environmental factors, or triggers, such as people, places, things, as well as anniversaries related to substance use and other behaviours associated with Addiction.

Post-traumatic stress disorder (PTSD). This condition may develop after a person is exposed to one or more traumatic events. The diagnosis may be given when a group of symptoms, such as disturbing recurring flashbacks, avoidance, or numbing of memories of the event, and hyperarousal continue for more than a month after the occurrence of a traumatic event.

Predisposition. The propensity towards having certain conditions. The term is usually used in the context of genetic predisposition, which refers to the genetic force that manifests certain health problems.

Prefrontal cortex (PFC). Located in the front of the brain, just behind the forehead, this is the part in charge of focus, forethought, impulse control, organization, empathy, and judgment; it is also responsible for regulating behaviour. The prefrontal cortex is a significant relay in the reward circuit and is modulated by dopamine.

Projection. Attribution of one's own ideas, feelings, or attitudes onto other people or objects. For example, viewing someone else as being blaming when you are the one feeling blame towards somebody, or cursing an object for falling on you and being clumsy when you feel responsible for being clumsy and knocking that object in the first place. Projection acts as a defense mechanism to protect us from uncomfortable feelings.

Psychoactive substance. A chemical substance that acts primarily upon the reward circuitry in the central nervous system resulting in a profound, usually immediate, change in perception and mood.

Psychoneuroimmunology. The study of the interaction of psychological or mental processes involving thoughts and feelings that affect the function of the nervous system, sometimes adversely. These processes can have related effects on the functioning of the immune system, resulting in illness.

Psychosis. A serious medical condition that reflects a disturbance in brain functioning. A person with psychosis experiences some loss of contact with reality, characterized by changes in their way of thinking, believing, perceiving, and/or behaving. For the person experiencing psychosis, the condition may not be perceived as pathological or be very disorienting or distressing. Without effective treatment, psychosis can overwhelm the lives of individuals and families.

Psychosocial. A combination of psychological and social factors.

Psychotherapy. Also called talk therapy, therapy, or counselling. Its purpose is the exploration of thoughts, feelings, and behaviour for the purpose of problem-solving or achieving higher levels of functioning and well-being. Technically speaking, counselling is the imparting of information or knowledge to an individual who does not have that knowledge, whereas therapy is the establishment of a relationship to understand the perspective of the individual experiencing problems and offers a dialogue to guide towards better coping and dealing with those problems more effectively.

Psychotropic substance. A chemical substance that acts primarily upon the central nervous system where it alters brain function, resulting in changes in perception, mood, consciousness and behaviour, usually over time. It may or may not be psychoactive.

Punishment. The provision of consequences that are primarily aversive, painful, or shaming in an effort to prevent that behaviour from occurring again. Punishment is typically not an effective way of preventing behaviour and reinforcement is a much more effective tool for behaviour change.

Qualitative. Descriptions or distinctions are based on a quality or characteristic rather than on a quantity or measured value.

Rationalization. Also known as making excuses, rationalization is a defense mechanism in which controversial behaviours or feelings are justified and explained in a seemingly rational or logical manner to avoid the true explanation.

Recovery. A process of sustained action that addresses the biological, psychological, social, and spiritual disturbances inherent in Addiction. Recovery aims to improve the quality of life by seeking balance and healing in all aspects of health and wellness, while addressing an individual's consistent pursuit of abstinence, impairment in behavioural control, dealing with cravings, recognizing problems in one's behaviours and interpersonal relationships, and dealing more effectively with emotional responses.

Reinforcer. A stimulus, such as a reward (positive reinforcement) or the removal of an unpleasant event (negative reinforcement) that maintains or strengthens a desired response.

Relapse. A process in which an individual who has established abstinence or sobriety experiences recurrence of signs and symptoms of active addiction, often including resumption of the pathological pursuit of reward and/or relief through the use of substances and other behaviours. When in relapse, there is often disengagement from recovery activities. Relapse can be triggered by exposure to: rewarding substances and behaviours, environmental cues to use, and emotional stressors that trigger heightened activity in brain stress circuits. The event of using or acting out is the latter part of the process, which can be prevented by early intervention.

Remission. A state of wellness where there is an abatement of signs and symptoms that characterize active Addiction. Many individuals in remission remain actively engaged in the process of recovery. Reduction in signs or symptoms constitutes improvement from a disease state, but remission involves a return to a level of functioning that is free of active symptoms and/or is marked by stability in the chronic signs and symptoms that characterize active Addiction.

Serenity. The state or quality of being serene, calm, or tranquil.

Sobriety. A state of sustained abstinence with a clear commitment to and active seeking of balance in the biological, psychological, social and spiritual aspects of an individual's health and wellness that were previously compromised by Addiction. It is the summation of abstinence in the context of recovery.

Solar plexus. Is a complex network of nerves (a plexus) located in the abdomen.

Stressors. Sources of stress, whether real or perceived.

Suboxone. Contains a combination of buprenorphine and naloxone. Suboxone is used to treat Addiction involving narcotics (opioids).

Substance abuse. Continued use despite harm due to lack of knowledge.

Substance dependence. Often considered synonymous with Addiction, it reflects continued use despite harm due to impaired control, craving, and compulsion.

Thalamus. A large, dual-lobed mass of gray matter buried under the cerebral cortex in the brain. It is involved in sensory perception and regulation of motor functions. The thalamus is a limbic system structure and it connects areas of the cerebral cortex that are involved in sensory perception and movement with other parts of the brain and spinal cord that also have a role in sensation and movement. As a regulator of sensory information, the thalamus also controls sleep and waking states of consciousness, while providing the ability to discriminate and choose among various processes or perceptions. It is associated with providing judgment in thought processes.

Triggers. Something that initiates a memory or reaction.

Ventral tegmental area (VTA). Located in the midbrain, at the top of the brainstem, the VTA is one of the most primitive parts of the brain. It is the neurons of the VTA that synthesize dopamine, which their axons then send to the nucleus accumbens. The VTA is also influenced by endorphins whose receptors are targeted by opiate drugs such as heroin and morphine.

Bibliography

Alcoholics Anonymous. (1939). *The Big Book*. New York: World Services, Inc.

Alcoholics Anonymous. (1988). *Twelve steps and twelve traditions* (38th ed.). New York: World Services, Inc.

Amen, D., & Smith, D. (2010). *Unchain your brain: 10 steps to breaking the addictions that steal your life*. Newport Beach, CA: Mindworks Press.

American Psychiatric Association (1980). *Diagnostic and statistical manual of mental disorders* (3rd ed.). Washington DC: American Psychiatric Publishing.

American Psychiatric Association (1987). *Diagnostic and statistical manual of mental disorders* (3rd ed. revised). Washington DC: American Psychiatric Publishing.

American Psychiatric Association (1994). *Diagnostic and statistical manual of mental disorders* (4th ed.). Washington DC: American Psychiatric Publishing.

American Psychiatric Association (2000). *Diagnostic and statistical manual of mental disorders* (4th ed. revised). Washington DC: American Psychiatric Publishing.

American Psychiatric Association (2013). *Diagnostic and statistical manual of mental disorders* (5th ed.). Washington DC: American Psychiatric Publishing.

American Society of Addiction Medicine (Adoption Date: April 12, 2011). Public Policy Statement: Definition of Addiction. www. ASAM.org

Barker, L. L., & Roach Gaut, D. (2002). *Communication* (8th ed.). Boston, MA: Pearson.

Beattie, M. (1992). *Codependent No More*. Center City, MN: Hazelden

Beck, J. S., & Beck, A. T. (2011). *Cognitive behaviour therapy: Basics and beyond* (2nd ed.). New York: Guilford Press.

Beck, A. T., Wright, F.D., Newman, C. F., & Liesen, B. S. (1993). *Cognitive therapy of substance abuse*. New York: Guilford Press.

Bell, R.G. (1970). *Escape from addiction*. New York, NY: McGraw-Hill Book Company.

Bell, R.G. (1989). *A special calling*. Toronto, ON: Stoddart Publishing Co. Limited.

Blum, K., Oscar-Berman M., Jacobs W., McLaughlin T., & Gold, M. (2014). Buprenorphine Response as a Function of Neurogenetic Polymorphic Antecedents: Can Dopamine Genes Affect Clinical Outcomes in Reward Deficiency Syndrome (RDS)? *Journal of Addiction Research Therapy*, 5: 185. Doi:10.4172/2155-6105.1000185.

Blum, K., Badgaiyan, R.D., Agan G., Fratantonio J., Simpatico T., et al. (2015). The Molecular Neurobiology of Twelve Steps Program & Fellowship: Connecting the Dots for Recovery. *Journal of Reward Deficiency Syndrome*, 1(1): 46-64.

Brown, B. (2007). *I thought it was just me (but it isn't): Making the journey from 'what will people think?' to 'I am enough.'* New York, NY: Penguin Group.

Brown, B. (2009). *Connections: A 12-session psychoeducational shame-resilience curriculum*. Center City, MN: Hazelden.

Brown, B. (2010). *The gifts of imperfection*. Center City, MN: Hazelden.

Doran, G. T. (1981). There's a S.M.A.R.T. way to write management's goals and objectives. *Management Review*, 70(11), 35–36.

DuPont, R. L. (2000). *The selfish brain: Learning from Addiction*. Center City, MN: Hazelden.

Edenberg, H. J. (2011, September 9). *Genetics of alcoholism*. Presented at the World Congress of Psychiatric Genetics symposium on The Genetics and Epigenetics of Substance Abuse. Presentation retrieved February 7, 2015 from http://www.drugabuse.gov/news-events/meetings-events/2011/09/genetics-epigenetics-substance-abuse

HBO Addiction Project (2007). www.drugabuse.gov/news-events/public/hbo-addiction-project. Retrieved July 14, 2014 from www.hbo.com

Karpman, S. (1968). Fairy tales and script drama analysis. *Transactional Analysis Bulletin*, 7 (26), 39-43.

Jellinek, E. M. (1960). *The Disease Concept of Alcoholism*. New Haven: Hillhouse.

Kendler, K. (2011, September 9). *The genetic epidemiology of substance abuse*. Presented at the World Congress of Psychiatric Genetics symposium on The Genetics and Epigenetics of Substance Abuse. Presentation retrieved February 7, 2015 from http://www.drugabuse.gov/news-events/meetings-events/2011/09/genetics-epigenetics-substance-abuse

Linehan, M. M. (2014). *Skills training manual for treating borderline personality disorder* (2nd ed.). New York: Guilford Press.

Luft, J., & Ingham, H. (1955). *The Johari window, a graphic model of interpersonal awareness*. Presented at the Proceedings of the Western Training Laboratory in Group Development. Retrieved

May 29, 2014 from http://www.businessballs.com/johariwin-dowmodel.htm

Mee-Lee, D. (Ed.). (2013). *The ASAM criteria: Treatment criteria for addictive, substance-related, and co-occurring conditions* (3rd ed.). Carson City, NV: The Change Companies.

Miller, W. R., & Rollnick, S. (2012). *Motivational interviewing: Helping people change* (3rd ed.). New York: Guilford Press.

Miller, W. R., & Rose, G. S. (2009). Toward a theory of motivational interviewing. *American Psychologist, 64*(6), 527-537.

Mooney, A. J., Dold, C. & Eisenberg H. (2014) *The Recovery Book: Answers to All Your Questions About Addiction and Alcoholism and Finding Health and Happiness in Sobriety* (2nd ed.). New York: Workman Publishing.

The National Center on Addiction and Substance Abuse (CASA). (2012). *CASA Columbia analysis of the National Survey on Drug Use and Health (NSDUH)*. Rockville, MD: U.S. Department of Health and Human Services, Substance Abuse and Mental Health Services Administration.

National Institute on Drug Abuse (n.d.). *Principles of drug abuse treatment for criminal justice populations: A research-based guide*. Retrieved February 6, 2015 from http://www.drugabuse.gov/sites/default/files/txcriminaljustice_0.pdf

National Institute on Drug Abuse (2014). *Drugs, brains and behaviour: The science of Addiction*. Retrieved February 7, 2015 from http://www.drugabuse.gov/sites/default/files/soa_2014.pdf

Nestler, E. (2011, September 9). *Epigenetics of addiction*. Presented at the World Congress of Psychiatric Genetics symposium on The Genetics and Epigenetics of Substance Abuse. Abstract retrieved February 7, 2015 from http://www.drugabuse.gov/news-events/meetings-events/2011/09/genetics-epigenetics-substance-abuse

Nicols, M. P. (2012). *Family therapy: Concepts and methods* (10ᵗʰ ed.). Upper Saddle River, NJ: Pearson Press.

Prochaska, J. O., & DiClemente, C. C. (2005). The transtheoretical approach. In J. C. Norcross, M. R. Goldfried (Eds.). *Handbook of psychotherapy integration* (2ⁿᵈ ed.) (pp. 147-171). New York: Oxford University Press.

Schaef, A. W. (1987). *When society becomes an addict.* New York, NY: Harper & Row.

Twerski, A. J. (1982). *It happens to doctors, too.* Center City, MN: Hazelden.

Twerski, A. J. (1997). *Addictive thinking: Understanding self-deception* (2ⁿᵈ ed.). Center City, MN: Hazelden.

Vaillant, G. (2005). Alcoholics Anonymous: Cult or cure? *Australian and New Zealand Journal of Psychiatry, 39,* 431-436.

Wegsheider-Cruse, S. (1986). *Choicemaking: For spirituality seekers, co-dependents and adult children.* Health Communications, Incorporated.

Yalom, I. (2002). *The gift of therapy: An open letter to a new generation of therapists and their patients.* New York: Harper Collins.

About the Authors

Dr. Raju Hajela is a principal of Health Upwardly Mobile Inc. (HUM) and the president and medical director. HUM was founded in 2009 as a health and wellness company in Calgary, Alberta, Canada, which specializes in Addiction, mental health, chronic pain and occupational health. Raju received his MD from Dalhousie University in 1982 and his Master of Public Health from the Harvard School of Public Health in 1988. Raju served in the Canadian Forces from 1979 to 1995. He has specialized training and extensive experience in Addiction, mental health, chronic pain, and occupational health. He has held leadership positions in provincial, national, and international medical organizations.

Ms. Sue Newton is a principal of Health Upwardly Mobile Inc. (HUM) and the vice president and operations director since its founding in 2009. She has been a registered nurse since 1988 and completed both her Bachelor of Arts degree in psychology and Bachelor of Science in nursing from Lakehead University in 1988. She received her master's degree in nursing from the University of Calgary in 1996. Sue initially worked for Alberta Health Services for nineteen years in both acute care and public health in a number of clinical and management roles. In 2008, she left Alberta Health Services to work as the nurse manager for an integrated health and wellness company in Calgary focusing on Occupational Health and employee and family health.

Ms. Paige Abbott is the clinical services director at Health Upwardly Mobile Inc. (HUM) and has been a member of the team since 2011. She completed her Master of Science degree in counselling psychology at the University of Calgary in 2007. She has been a Registered Psychologist in Alberta since 2009. After graduation, Paige worked at an employee and family assistance program (EFAP) from 2008-2012 where she worked with a broad range of issues, including Addiction and mental health. She also has experience volunteering with marginalized populations and has been involved in research on topics such as spirituality, HIV/AIDS, and homeless street youth.